Manual of Normative Measurements in Head and Neck Imaging

T0171898

Daniel Thomas Ginat
Editor

Manual of Normative Measurements in Head and Neck Imaging

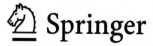 Springer

Editor
Daniel Thomas Ginat
Department of Radiology
University of Chicago
Chicago, IL
USA

ISBN 978-3-030-50566-0   ISBN 978-3-030-50567-7   (eBook)
https://doi.org/10.1007/978-3-030-50567-7

This Springer imprint is published by the registered company Springer Nature Switzerland AG
The registered company address is: Gewerbestrasse 11, 6330 Cham, Switzerland

Foreword

The head and neck region is considered as one of the most complex anatomical parts of the body. Therefore, many radiologists have concerns reading CT and MRIs of the head and neck region. The chapters of this *Manual of Normative Measurements in Head and Neck Imaging* will aid you in the interpretation of scans with excellent image examples and informative measurement technique. The book is conveniently divided by body regions, ranging from the orbit, the most complex region the temporal bone with its narrow anatomical landmarks, the skull base, cervical lymph nodes, and the salivary glands. All of these topics are extensively discussed.

Correct measurements of anatomical landmarks are crucial to discriminate normal variants from pathological conditions. Moreover, it is of crucial importance for every radiologist to be familiar with the correct measurement and localization of lymph nodes according to the established level classification. In clinical work, some common mistakes such as incorrect measurements, e.g., to measure the long axis, can lead to false radiology report and could also lead to wrong treatment of the patients. Notably, to report the lymph node levels is important for communicating with clinicians.

To conclude, this book can be recommended as a companion at the workplace of every radiologist to look up the measurements of the landmarks and to correctly assess the complex head and neck region.

Alexey Surov
Department of Radiology and Nuclear Medicine
Otto-von-Guericke University,
Magdeburg, Germany

Preface

When it comes to evaluating many structures on radiology images, size matters! This book is intended to serve as a useful and concise reference for making and interpreting anatomic measurements on head and neck imaging. Normative data are compiled and organized based on the following subregions of the head and neck: orbits, temporal bones, skull base, craniocervical junction, lymph nodes, and thyroid, salivary glands, and tonsillar tissues. In particular, imaging examples of normal measurements and relevant abnormalities are illustrated. It is important to keep in mind that the reference measurements presented in this text are only to be used as a general guide and that interpreting imaging often requires considering other factors than just size.

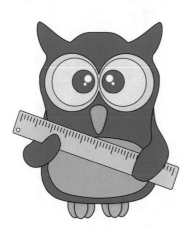

Chicago, IL, USA   Daniel Thomas Ginat

Contents

Basic Quantitative Imaging Approaches

1

Daniel Thomas Ginat

1.1 Line and Angle Measurements

A typical picture archive and communication system (PACS) image viewer offers a basic palette of measurements, including the commonly used line and angle functions (Fig. 1.1), which can be drawn manually by the user on the images of interest.

Measurements are typically made using the metric system. It should be cautioned that systems that display line and angle measurements to one-tenth of a millimeter or degree do not actually have the accuracy to justify so many significant digits. Another pitfall regarding line measurements on cross-sectional imaging is that these can be affected by variations in the patient positioning (Fig. 1.2). This issue can be mitigated by implementing the standard positioning of patients in scanners or reformatting the images such that they are consistent between exams.

Most anatomic structures in the population have a normal distribution of size. Reference normative measurements available in the literature and in the subsequent chapters in this book are often

D. T. Ginat (✉)
Department of Radiology, Section of Neuroradiology,
University of Chicago, Chicago, IL, USA
e-mail: dtg1@uchicago.edu

© Springer Nature Switzerland AG 2021
D. T. Ginat (ed.), *Manual of Normative Measurements in Head and Neck Imaging*, https://doi.org/10.1007/978-3-030-50567-7_1

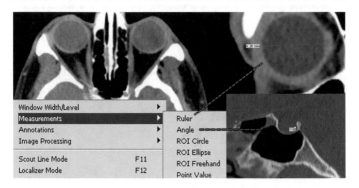

Fig. 1.1 Screenshot of the measurement palette on PACS with example ruler and angle markers

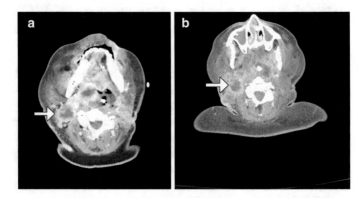

Fig. 1.2 Sequential computed tomography (CT) images (**a** and **b**) at the level of a necrotic right cervical lymph node (arrows) show differences in angulation of the patient, in which the lesion is at the level of the maxillary sinuses on one image and at the level of the teeth on the other image

reported as averages of sample populations, sometimes along with standard deviations, ranges, or 95% confidence intervals (CI), which quantify the degree of variation that measurements have within a sample population. These statistical parameters can be used as guidelines to help decide whether measurements obtained on particular scans are normal or abnormal.

1.2   Area and Volume Measurements

For many clinical applications, size is better represented in terms of cross-sectional areas and volumes than unidimensional measurements, especially for structures with an irregular shape. There are several techniques for determining volume on imaging, including the following:

- The prorate ellipsoid formulas for the cross-sectional area and volume:

$$\text{Area} = \pi \times \text{length} \times \text{width}$$

$$\text{Volume} = 0.52 \times \text{height} \times \text{length} \times \text{width}$$

  Although straightforward, these formulas can be less accurate if the shape deviates substantially from a circle or sphere.

- Planimetry is a more reliable, but more time-consuming, method for measuring volume in which the edge of the structure is traced on all image slices and cross-sectional areas are summed and multiplied by the slice thickness.

- Specialized software can be used to recognize the edges of structures, for example, using threshold-based, connected components, or region-growing algorithms, to segment an organ or lesion and thereby automate determination of volumes (Fig. 1.3).

In general, thin slice reconstructions of 1 mm or at least no more than 3 mm are recommended for reliable volume measurements on cross-sectional imaging.

1.3   CT Attenuation and MRI Signal Intensity Measurements

In addition to measuring the size of a structure, the value of the pixel intensity can be ascertained. This can be accomplished by drawing a region of interest on the image. On computed

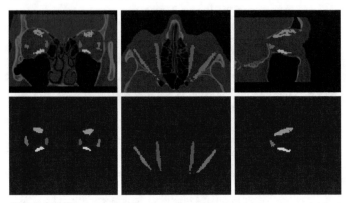

Volume (mm3)
Medial rectus, Lateral, Superior (+Superior Levator Palpabrae), Inferior rectus
2177, 1888, 2453, 1660

Fig. 1.3 Volume measurements of the extraocular muscles generated using machine learning automatic segmentation. Courtesy of Ramkumar Rajabathar Babu Jai Shanker

tomography (CT), the region of interest can provide measurement of attenuation via Hounsfield units (HU). Different tissues and materials have characteristic attenuation values (Fig. 1.4). On magnetic resonance imaging (MRI), T1- and T2-weighted signal intensity can also be measured using regions of interest, as well as the diffusivity of protons on apparent diffusion coefficient (ADC) maps derived from diffusion-weighted imaging (Fig. 1.5).

1.4   Measurement Errors

There are three main types of measurement errors: systematic errors, random errors, and gross errors:

- Systematic errors lead to inaccurate measurements that trend in one direction and occur due to fault in the measuring device, including scanners. This can manifest with partial volume averaging, in which the computed tomography (CT) attenuation

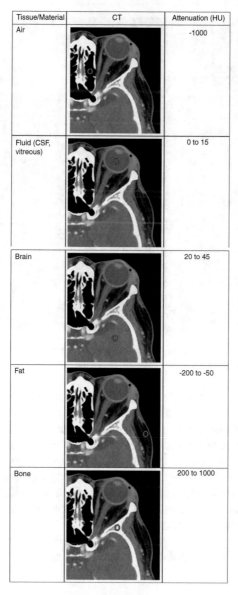

Fig. 1.4 Schematic showing the typical attenuation values of different materials and tissues on computed tomography (CT)

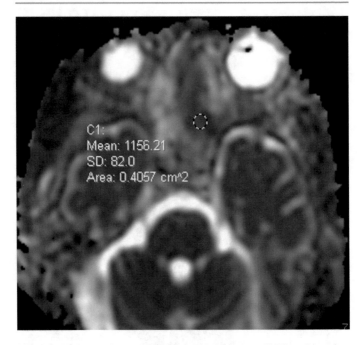

Fig. 1.5 ADC map shows a diffusion region of interest (ROI) positioned on a left sinonasal tumor

or MRI signal of a structure within a voxel blends with other structures. This is particularly noticeable between low versus high magnification images. At low magnification, the edges of certain structures can appear rather distinct, but at increasing degrees of magnification, the edge is actually blurry (Fig. 1.6). The width of this gray zone is particularly significant relative to structures of submillimeter size, which can render the measurement inaccurate. Such issues can be mitigated by using ultrathin-section acquisition.

- Random errors lead to inconsistent variations in measurement. This can be attributable to the inherent noise in images

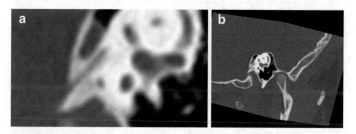

Fig. 1.6 Sagittal oblique computed tomography (CT) images without (**a**) and with (**b**) magnification show that the anatomical margins become blurred with magnification

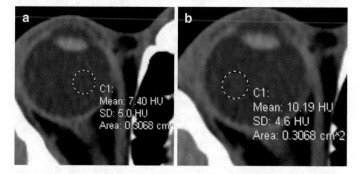

Fig. 1.7 Axial computed tomography (CT) images (**a** and **b**) show the different attenuation measurements of the globe contents at slightly different positions due to noise, each with substantial standard deviations

(Fig. 1.7) and factors such as intraobserver and interobserver variability, whereby the same individual will obtain different measurements of the same thing at different times or different individuals will obtain different measurements of the same thing.

• Gross errors are those in which the wrong measurement is recorded, such as entering 18 mm instead of 13 mm, for example.

Further Reading

Abramson RG, Burton KR, Yu JP, Scalzetti EM, Yankeelov TE, Rosenkrantz AB, Mendiratta-Lala M, Bartholmai BJ, Ganeshan D, Lenchik L, Subramaniam RM. Methods and challenges in quantitative imaging biomarker development. Acad Radiol. 2015;22(1):25–32.

Buerke B, Puesken M, Beyer F, et al. Semiautomatic lymph node segmentation in multislice computed tomography: impact of slice thickness on segmentation quality, measurement precision, and interobserver variability. Invest Radiol. 2010;45(2):82–8.

Dejaco D, Url C, Schartinger VH, et al. Approximation of head and neck cancer volumes in contrast enhanced CT. Cancer Imaging. 2015;15:16. Published 2015 Sep 29.

Fabel M, Wulff A, Heckel F, et al. Clinical lymph node staging—influence of slice thickness and reconstruction kernel on volumetry and RECIST measurements. Eur J Radiol. 2012;81(11):3124–30.

Fehlings MG, Furlan JC, Massicotte EM, et al. Interobserver and intraobserver reliability of maximum canal compromise and spinal cord compression for evaluation of acute traumatic cervical spinal cord injury. Spine (Phila Pa 1976). 2006;31(15):1719–25.

Ginat DT, Gupta R. Advances in computed tomography imaging technology. Annu Rev Biomed Eng. 2014;16:431–53.

Juliano AF, Ting EY, Mingkwansook V, Hamberg LM, Curtin HD. Vestibular aqueduct measurements in the 45° oblique (Pöschl) plane. AJNR Am J Neuroradiol. 2016;37(7):1331–7.

Mueller S, Wichmann G, Dornheim L, et al. Different approaches to volume assessment of lymph nodes in computer tomography scans of head and neck squamous cell carcinoma in comparison with a real gold standard. ANZ J Surg. 2012;82(10):737–41.

Rosenkrantz AB, Mendiratta-Lala M, Bartholmai BJ, Ganeshan D, Abramson RG, Burton KR, Yu JP, Scalzetti EM, Yankeelov TE, Subramaniam RM, Lenchik L. Clinical utility of quantitative imaging. Acad Radiol. 2015;22(1):33–49.

Wilson JD, Eardley W, Odak S, Jennings A. To what degree is digital imaging reliable? Validation of femoral neck shaft angle measurement in the era of picture archiving and communication systems. Br J Radiol. 2011;84(1000):375–9.

Zhu W, Huang Y, Zeng L, et al. AnatomyNet: deep learning for fast and fully automated whole-volume segmentation of head and neck anatomy. Med Phys. 2019;46(2):576–89.

Normative Measurements of Orbital Walls and Contents

2

Mathew B. Macey, Juan E. Small, and Daniel Thomas Ginat

2.1   Orbital Walls

Each orbit is surrounded by medial, superior, lateral, and inferior orbital walls, which have a pyramidal configuration with the apex posteriorly. Several anatomical landmarks can be used to ascertain the separation between the two orbits (Fig. 2.1).

Interorbital distance (measured at the posterior border of the frontal processes of the maxilla in the plane of the optic nerve):

- At birth: 14.2 ± 0.7 mm
- At 1 year: 16.2 ± 0.8 mm

M. B. Macey
New York Institute of Technology College of Osteopathic Medicine, Old Westbury, NY, USA

J. E. Small
Department of Radiology, Section of Neuroradiology, Lahey Hospital and Medical Center, Burlington, MA, USA

D. T. Ginat (✉)
Department of Radiology, Section of Neuroradiology, University of Chicago, Chicago, IL, USA
e-mail: dtg1@uchicago.edu

© Springer Nature Switzerland AG 2021
D. T. Ginat (ed.), *Manual of Normative Measurements in Head and Neck Imaging*, https://doi.org/10.1007/978-3-030-50567-7_2

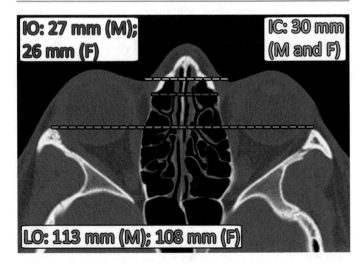

Fig. 2.1 Interorbital (IO), intercanthal (IC), and lateral orbital (LO) distances. Axial computed tomography (CT) image shows the typical measurements for adult males (M) and females (F)

- Adult males: 27 mm (range: 23–32 mm)
- Adult females: 26 mm (range: 23–32 mm)

The normal interorbital distance measured at the posterior border of the frontal processes of the maxilla on nonrotated scans, in the plane of the optic nerve, ranges from 23 to 32 mm (average: 27 mm) in men and 23 to 32 mm (average: 26 mm) in women. The widest interorbital (IO) distance lies behind the posterior poles of the globes. This ranges from 32 to 41 mm (average: 34 mm) in men and 29 to 37 mm (average: 32 mm) in women.

Inner intercanthal (IC) distance (measured between the medial canthi):

- At birth: 22 ± 1 mm
- At 1 year: 28 ± 1 mm
- Adult male: 30 mm (range: 27–35 mm)
- Adult female: 30 mm (range: 25–33 mm)

Lateral orbital (LO) distance (measured between the lateral orbital rims):

- Average at birth: 66 ± 2 mm
- Average at 1 year: 78 ± 2 mm
- Adult male average: 113 mm (range: 105–120 mm)
- Adult female average: 108 mm (range: 98–115 mm)

Practical implications: Normal measurements of orbital relationships are a useful reference for evaluating hypo- and hypertelorism associated with craniofacial abnormalities and surgical reconstruction. Measurements are most reliable based on images in the Frankfort horizontal plane, which joins the anthropometric landmarks of porion and orbitale (Fig. 2.2).

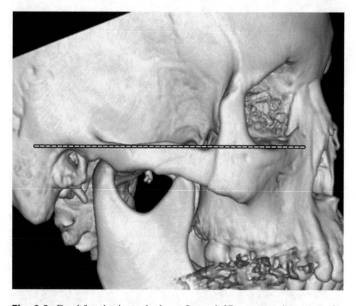

Fig. 2.2 Frankfort horizontal plane. Lateral 3D computed tomography (CT) image shows the orientation of the Frankfort horizontal plane, which extends from the superior aspect of the external auditory canal to the inferior orbital rim

Lateral Wall:

- The lateral orbital wall is formed by the greater wing of the sphenoid, frontal, and zygomatic bones.
- The deep lateral orbital wall comprises the sphenoid trigone, which has a triangular configuration on axial images.
- The typical distance of the lateral orbital rim to the apex is 35–40 mm in adults (Fig. 2.3).
- The average distance from the lateral orbital rim to the point where the lateral rectus muscle contacted the bone is 25–26 mm.

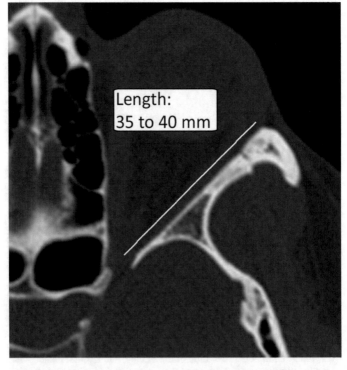

Fig. 2.3 Lateral orbital wall. Axial computed tomography (CT) image shows the average distance from the lateral orbital rim to the orbital apex

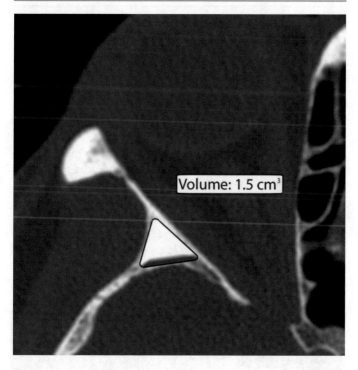

Fig. 2.4 Sphenoid trigone. Axial computed tomography (CT) image shows the overall sphenoid trigone volume

- The average width of the lateral wall at the level of the superior border of the lateral rectus muscle at the thickest part on the coronal image is 16 mm.
- The sphenoid trigone has an average volume of 1.5 cm^3 (Fig. 2.4).

Practical implications: The deep lateral orbital wall is considered an effective and safe site for orbital decompression surgery. The degree of lateral decompression is dependent on the volume of the sphenoid trigone comprising the deep lateral orbital wall. The width and length of the thickest segment of the greater wing of the sphenoid can be used as anatomic guidelines during deep lateral orbital decompression surgery.

Medial Wall:

- The distance of the medial orbital rim to the apex is approximately 45 mm.
- The anterior ethmoid foramen, which contains the anterior ethmoidal artery, is located approximately 15 mm posterior to the medial orbital rim at the level of the junction of the frontal bone with the ethmoid bone (Fig. 2.5).
- Approximately 12 mm more posteriorly is the posterior ethmoid foramen through which the posterior ethmoidal artery passes.

Practical implications: The ethmoid arteries can be the source of epistaxis and orbital hemorrhage. Therefore, it is important to have a sense of where these are located for surgery in the medial orbital wall region.

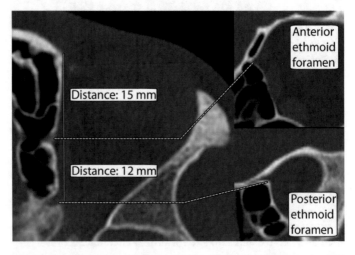

Fig. 2.5   Medial orbital wall. Axial and coronal computed tomography (CT) images depict the typical location of the anterior and posterior ethmoid foramina along the medial orbital wall

Inferior Orbital (Sphenomaxillary) Fissure:

- The inferior orbital fissure is located in the orbital floor adjacent to the superior orbital fissure, foramen rotundum, pterygopalatine fossa, infratemporal fossa, and temporal fossa.
- Bounded by the lower margin of the orbital surface of the greater wing of the sphenoid, laterally by the zygoma, posteromedially by the orbital process of the palatine bone, and anteriorly by the maxilla.
- Transmits the infraorbital nerve and artery.
- Oriented in an anterolateral direction from the maxillary strut posteriorly to the zygomatic bone anteriorly.
- Narrower at its center and its long axis lies along the line between the zygomaticofacial foramen and the optic canal.
- The average length of the inferior orbital fissure is 29 mm, with a range of 25–35 mm (Fig. 2.6).

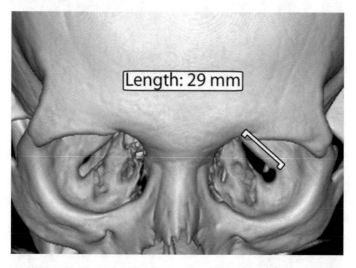

Fig. 2.6 Inferior orbital fissure. 3D computed tomography (CT) image shows the typical length of the inferior orbital fissure

Practical implications: The inferior orbital fissure is an important anatomic landmark for endonasal endoscopic approaches to the skull base and orbit.

Infraorbital Nerve Canal:

- The infraorbital nerve canal transmits the infraorbital nerve, which is the termination of the maxillary nerve and provides sensory function.
- The nerve exits the skull through the foramen rotundum and enters into the pterygopalatine fossa. It then enters the infraorbital groove and passes through the infraorbital canal. The nerve emerges in front of the maxilla through the infraorbital foramen.
- The mean infraorbital foramen to infraorbital margin distance is 7 ± 1 mm (Fig. 2.7).

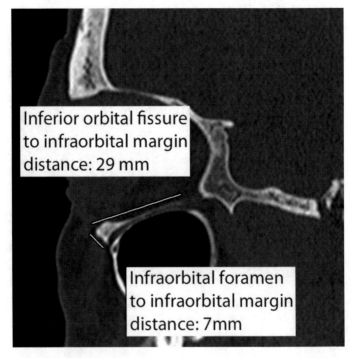

Inferior orbital fissure to infraorbital margin distance: 29 mm

Infraorbital foramen to infraorbital margin distance: 7mm

Fig. 2.7 Infraorbital canal. Sagittal computed tomography (CT) image shows the relation of the infraorbital nerve to neighboring landmarks

- The distance from the inferior orbital fissure to the infraorbital margin is 29 ± 2 mm.

Practical implications: The infraorbital nerve is at risk for iatrogenic injury during orbital floor repair.

2.2   Globe

- The globe occupies one-third of the overall orbital volume and consists of the outer wall, anterior chamber, lens, and vitreous body.
- The wall of the globe comprises three layers: the outer fibrous coat (sclera and cornea), the uvea (iris, ciliary body, and choroid), and the retina.
- The full-term newborn globe mean axial length is 16–18 mm.
- The globe (axial length) tends to grow until 16–18 years of age. Axial length, anterior chamber depth, and vitreous chamber depth then decrease with age, while lens thickness increases with age.
- Growth of the globe stops within 1 year after birth, with a mean globe diameter of 23 mm (range: 22–25 mm) (Fig. 2.8).
- The normal position of the posterior margin of the globe on axial CT images is 9–10 mm posterior to the interzygomatic line on average (range: 6–13 mm).
- The sclera measures up to 1 mm in thickness and appears hypointense on magnetic resonance imaging (MRI).
- The cornea is a component of the refractive system and measures 0.5 mm in thickness centrally. On MRI, the cornea is a low signal intensity convex structure due to the collagen content.
- The average depth of the normal anterior chamber is about 2.5 mm, but ranges from 1.5 to 4 mm depending on demographics (Fig. 2.9).
- The lens is an ovoid crystalline structure that forms the posterior boundary of the anterior chamber and is attached to the ciliary body via the zonular fibers. The lens displays low signal on both T1- and T2-weighted sequences and typically measures 5 mm in anteroposterior thickness and 9 mm in equatorial length (Fig. 2.10).

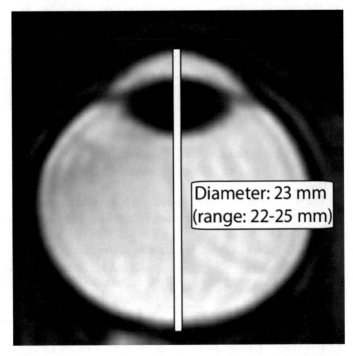

Fig. 2.8 Overall globe dimensions. Axial T2-weighted magnetic resonance imaging (MRI) shows the typical width and range of the adult globe diameter

- The vitreous humor comprises two-thirds of the volume of the globe.
- The posterior walls of the globes are typically 9–10 mm posterior to the interzygomatic line (Fig. 2.11).

Practical implications: The size of the globe is relevant for diagnosing buphthalmos or microphthalmos (Fig. 2.12). MRI ocular volumetry measurement error rates with RARE are lower than with FSPGR sequences. Fast spin echo (FSE) images acquired with fat suppression minimize chemical shift artifact in the region of the sclera. In any patient, a discrepancy on CT

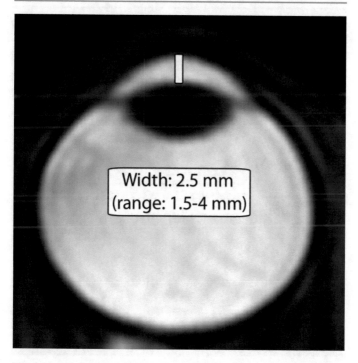

Fig. 2.9 Anterior chamber. Axial T2-weighted magnetic resonance imaging (MRI) shows the typical width and range of the normal adult anterior chamber

images of 2 mm or more between the depths of the anterior chambers of the normal and abnormal eyes or a depth measuring over 5 mm raises the possibility of scleral rupture (Fig. 2.13).

2.3   Optic Nerve and Sheath

The optic nerve is an extension of white matter tracts from the retina to the brain and is surrounded by cerebrospinal fluid that is continuous with the intracranial subarachnoid space. In turn, the

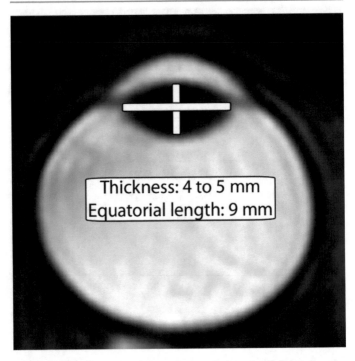

Fig. 2.10 Lens. Axial T2-weighted magnetic resonance imaging (MRI) shows the average dimensions of the adult lens

optic nerve sheath is a layer of dura that surrounds the optic nerve and cerebrospinal fluid. The optic nerve sheath can vary in width with changes in cerebrospinal fluid pressure.

- *Optic Nerve Width*:
  - Normal pediatric optic nerve diameters measured 10 mm posterior to the optic disk are listed in Table 2.1.
  - A lower bound to the 95% prediction interval for normal optic nerves is (2.24 mm + 0.05 × [age in years]) mm.
  - Adult optic nerve diameter declines from the anterior to posterior orbit and measures 4.0 mm just posterior to the

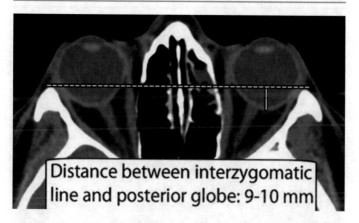

Fig. 2.11 Proptosis measurement. Axial computed tomography (CT) image denotes the typical normal position of the globe with respect to the interzygomatic line

globe and 3.5 mm at 10 mm posterior to the globe (Fig. 2.14).

- *Optic Nerve Length*:
  - Intraocular segment: 1 mm—emerges through the scleral opening
  - Intraorbital segment: 25 mm—the longest segment and the communication between subarachnoid space around the optic nerve with that in suprasellar cistern
  - Canalicular segment: 9 mm
- *Optic Nerve Sheath*:
  - Children, measured 10 mm anterior to the optic foramen on axial T2 sequence:
    - 0–3 years: 3.1 mm
    - 3–6 years: 4.1 mm
    - 6–18 years: 3.6 mm

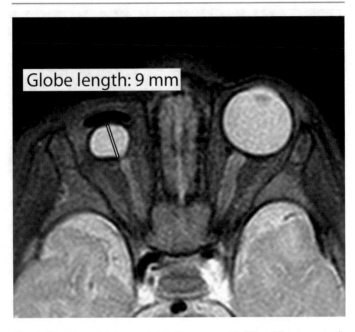

Fig. 2.12 Microphthalmos. Axial fat-suppressed T2-weighted magnetic resonance imaging (MRI) shows a small right globe

- Adults: The optic nerve sheath diameters on CT are 4.9–5.2 ± 1.3–1.5 mm at 3 mm, 4.4–4.5 ± 0.6–0.8 mm at 8 mm from the globe, and 3.6–3.7 ± 0.7–0.8 mm at 3 mm from the optic canal (Fig. 2.15).
- Normal values of the optic nerve sheath complex on CT (mean ± 2 SDs) at the retrobulbar and waist regions are 5.6 ± 1.8 (3.8–7.4) mm and 3.7 ± 0.8 (2.9–4.5) mm, respectively.
- There is no correlation between age, gender, and size of the optic nerve sheath complex.

Practical implications: The least variable results are obtained 8–10 mm posterior to the globe. The optic nerve diameter is smaller in glaucoma patients but larger in patients with increased intracranial pressure. The anatomic extension of the subarachnoid

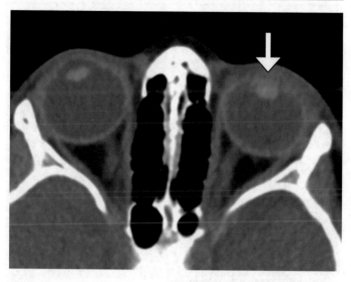

Fig. 2.13 Globe rupture. Axial computed tomography (CT) image shows collapse of the left anterior chamber (arrow) in a child who was stabbed in the eye with scissors

Table 2.1 Normal pediatric optic nerve diameters measured 10 mm posterior to the optic disk

Age (year)	Diameter (mm)
0–1.5	2.2
1.5–3	2.4
3–6	2.6
6–12	2.9
12–18	3.1

space underneath the optic nerve sheath is thought to be responsible for the transmission of these forces. Conditions in which the optic nerve sheath complex can be enlarged include neoplasms, such as gliomas (Fig. 2.16), pseudotumor, cerebri, infection, hemorrhage, and acute optic neuritis. The optic nerve sheath complex can be abnormally small in cases of chronic ischemia or septo-optic dysplasia.

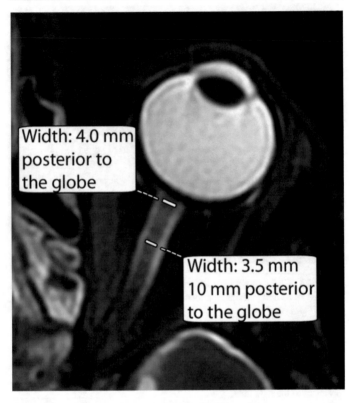

Fig. 2.14 Optic nerve. Axial T2-weighted magnetic resonance imaging (MRI) shows the typical widths of the optic nerve in an adult

2.4 Extraocular Muscles

- The extraocular muscles that are responsible for moving the globe include the superior, inferior, medial, and lateral recti and the superior and inferior oblique muscles.
- The levator palpebrae superioris is responsible for moving the superior eyelid.
- The normal sizes of the extraocular muscles in adults are listed in Table 2.2 and shown in Fig. 2.17.

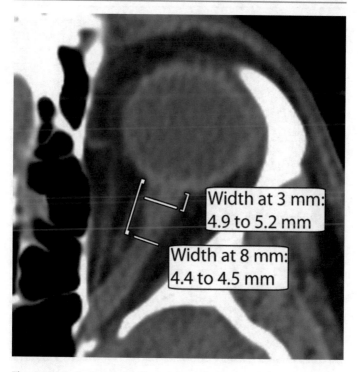

Fig. 2.15 Optic nerve sheath. Axial computed tomography (CT) image shows that the optic nerve sheath is typically wider just posterior to the globe versus more posteriorly

- All extraocular recti muscles increase in thickness from childhood, with the most dramatic growth occurring in the first 5–6 months of life. This growth continues as outlined in Table 2.2, until about 60 years old when the thickness begins to decline.
- The inferior rectus and superior group muscles are measured in the coronal plane, while the medal and lateral rectus muscles can be measured on the axial or coronal planes, but the coronal plane measurements tend to be 1.5 and 1.2 times

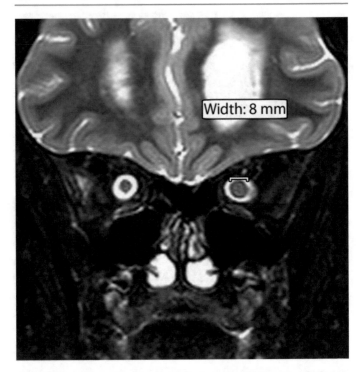

Fig. 2.16 Optic glioma. Coronal T2-weighted magnetic resonance imaging (MRI) shows enlargement of the left orbital optic nerve. There is also dilatation of the bilateral optic nerve sheaths and partly imaged dilatation of the left lateral ventricle in a patient with neurofibromatosis type 1

Table 2.2 Normal dimensions of the extraocular muscles in adults

Extraocular muscle	Maximum cross-sectional thickness (mm)	Maximum cross-sectional area (mm²)
Medial rectus	3.5–4.2	27.9–30.3
Lateral rectus	3.2–3.3	32.2–41.2
Inferior rectus	4.2–4.8	28.0–33.6
Superior group[a]	3.9–4.6	33.0–34.4
Superior oblique	–	13.8–19.0
Inferior oblique	1.5–2.8	21.6

[a]Since they cannot be reliably distinguished from each other, the superior rectus and the levator palpebrae superior muscles are measured together

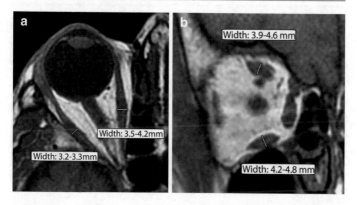

Fig. 2.17 Extraocular muscles. Axial (**a**) and coronal (**b**) T1-weighted MR images show the typical widths of the horizontal and vertical extraocular muscles

greater than the axial plane measurement for these muscles, respectively.

Practical implications: The mean diameters of the extraocular muscles in males are significantly larger than in females. Total extraocular muscle volume is not conserved, but actually increases with contraction and decreases with relaxation. Owing to the dramatic postnatal changes in extraocular muscle size and insertional position, it is generally safer to perform extraocular muscle surgery after about 6 months of age. Enlargement of the extraocular muscles, particularly the inferior, medial, and superior rectus muscles, can be a manifestation of thyroid eye disease (Fig. 2.18). Since denervated extraocular muscles do not readily atrophy, abnormally small muscles may be a sign of chronic progressive external ophthalmoplegia. Other conditions that can result in extraocular muscle enlargement include contusion, infection, and neoplasm.

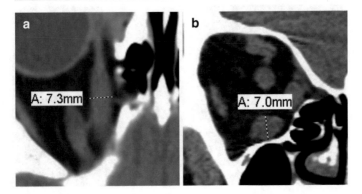

Fig. 2.18 Thyroid eye disease. Axial (**a**) and coronal (**b**) computed tomography (CT) images show enlargement of multiple right inferior and medial rectus muscles

2.5   Lacrimal Gland

- The lacrimal gland produces the aqueous portion of the tear film and is located in the anterior, superotemporal orbit within the lacrimal fossa of the frontal bone.
- Secretions are emptied into a duct system that delivers the fluid to the ocular surface. The outflow component of the lacrimal system lies at the nasal side of the eye, where puncta located on the upper and lower lids drain fluid into canaliculi that lead to the nasolacrimal sac and nasal cavity.
- The lacrimal gland can have a bilobed shape due to indentation by the levator palpebrae superioris tendon, with a small palpebral component underneath the eyelid and a larger orbital component.
- The average dimensions of the lacrimal gland are as follows (Fig. 2.19):
    - Axial width: 5 mm
    - Axial length: 15 mm
    - Coronal height: 20 mm

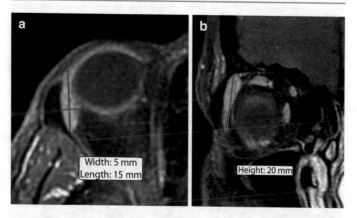

Fig. 2.19 Lacrimal gland. Axial (**a**) and coronal (**b**) post-contrast T1-weighted MR images show the typical dimensions of the normal lacrimal gland

- The mean volume for lacrimal glands in adults ranges from 0.7 to 0.8 cm^3.

Practical implications: Lacrimal gland volume and dimensions decrease with age, but there is no significant variation with gender or laterality. Lacrimal gland measurements may differ between ethnicities. Lacrimal glands in the patients with Sjögren syndrome can be hypertrophic, normal in size, or atrophic. Accelerated fat deposition can be detected with MR imaging and can be a distinctive feature of lacrimal glands that are affected by Sjögren's syndrome. A significant increase in lacrimal gland volume can be seen in thyroid-associated ophthalmopathy patients. The lacrimal gland can also be diffusely enlarged in other conditions, including sarcoidosis, orbital inflammation, and neoplasms, such as lymphoma (Fig. 2.20).

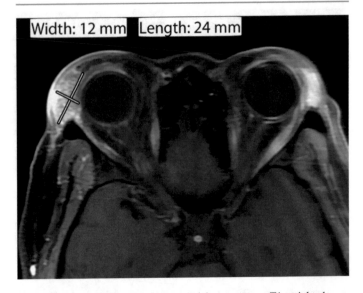

Fig. 2.20 Lacrimal gland lymphoma. Axial post-contrast T1-weighted magnetic resonance imaging (MRI) shows asymmetric diffuse enlargement of the right lacrimal gland

2.6   Superior Ophthalmic Vein

- The superior ophthalmic vein typically originates from the junction of the supraorbital and angular veins, approximately 4–5 mm posterior to the superior oblique tendon.
- The superior ophthalmic vein joins the inferior ophthalmic vein and passes through the superior orbital fissure.
- The superior ophthalmic vein consistently runs lateral to the ophthalmic artery, but has an asymmetric outer diameter bilaterally. The mean outer diameter at the crossing point is 1.6–1.7 mm (Fig. 2.21).

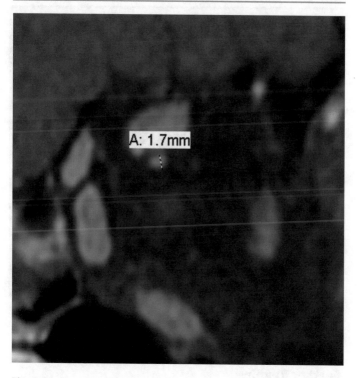

Fig. 2.21 Superior ophthalmic vein. Coronal post-contrast fat-suppressed T1-weighted magnetic resonance imaging (MRI) shows the typical dimension of the vessel

Practical implications: Enlargement of the superior ophthalmic vein can be associated with carotid-cavernous fistulas, arteriovenous malformations, thrombosis, compression, thyroid eye disease, orbital pseudotumors, retrocavernous tumors, elevated intracranial pressure, and intubation (Fig. 2.22). A diameter of ≥2 mm on axial CT scans is a possible indicator of enlargement, diameter ≥3 mm is likely to be an indicator, and diameter ≥4 mm is a definite indicator.

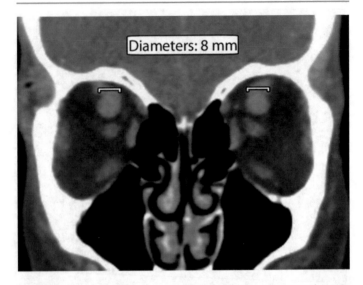

Fig. 2.22 Superior ophthalmic vein enlargement. Coronal computed tomography (CT) image shows the superior ophthalmic veins are significantly enlarged bilaterally in a patient with congestive heart failure and intubation

Further Reading

Ankur G, Xin Z. Lacrimal gland development: from signaling interactions to regenerative medicine. Dev Dyn. 2017;246(12):970–80.

Bingham CM, Castro A, Realini T, Nguyen J, Hogg JP, Sivak-Callcott JA. Calculated CT volumes of lacrimal glands in normal Caucasian orbits. Ophthalmic Plast Reconstr Surg. 2013;29(3):157–9.

Bourlet P, Carrie D, Garcier JM, Dalens H, Chansolme D, Viallet JF, Boyer L. Study of the inferior oblique muscle of the eye by MRI. Surg Radiol Anat. 1998;20(2):119–21.

Bukhari AA, Basheer NA, Joharjy HI. Age, gender, and interracial variability of normal lacrimal gland volume using MRI. Ophthalmic Plast Reconstr Surg. 2014;30(5):388–91.

Carlow TJ, Depper MH, Orrison WW Jr. MR of extraocular muscles in chronic progressive external ophthalmoplegia. AJNR Am J Neuroradiol. 1998;19(1):95–9.

Clark RA, Demer JL. Changes in extraocular muscle volume during ocular duction. Invest Ophthalmol Vis Sci. 2016;57(3):1106–11.

De Battista JC, Zimmer LA, Theodosopoulos PV, Froelich SC, Keller JT. Anatomy of the inferior orbital fissure: implications for endoscopic cranial base surgery. J Neurol Surg B Skull Base. 2012;73(2):132–8.

Elhadi AM, Zaidi HA, Yagmurlu K, Ahmed S, Rhoton AL Jr, Nakaji P, Preul MC, Little AS. Infraorbital nerve: a surgically relevant landmark for the pterygopalatine fossa, cavernous sinus, and anterolateral skull base in endoscopic transmaxillary approaches. J Neurosurg. 2016;125(6):1460–8.

Erdogan B, Alper Y, Bahar Y, Hasmet Y, Gulen D. Evaluation of lacrimal gland dimensions and volume in Turkish population with computed tomography. J Clin Diagn Res. 2016;10(2):TC06–8.

Hallinan JT, Pillay P, Koh LH, Goh KY, Yu WY. Eye globe abnormalities on MR and CT in adults: an anatomical approach. Korean J Radiol. 2016;17(5):664–73.

Hashemi H, Khabazkhoob M, Miraftab M, Emamian MH, Shariati M, Abdolahinia T, Fotouhi A. The distribution of axial length, anterior chamber depth, lens thickness, and vitreous chamber depth in an adult population of Shahroud, Iran. BMC Ophthalmol. 2012;12:50.

Hashemi H, Jafarzadehpur E, Ghaderi S, Yekta A, Ostadimoghaddam H, Norouzirad R, Khabazkhoob M. Ocular components during the ages of ocular development. Acta Ophthalmol. 2015;93(1):e74–81.

Huanmanop T, Agthong S, Chentanez V. Surgical anatomy of fissures and foramina in the orbits of Thai adults. J Med Assoc Thail. 2007;90(11):2383–91.

Hyoun-Do H, Ji-Hye K, Seong-Jae K, Ji-Myong Y, Seong-Wook S. The change of lacrimal gland volume in Korean patients with thyroid-associated ophthalmopathy. Korean J Ophthalmol. 2016;30(5):319–25.

Izumi M, Eguchi K, Uetani M, Nakamura H, Takagi Y, Hayashi K, et al. MR features of the lacrimal gland in Sjögren's syndrome. Am J Roentgenol. 1998;170:1661–6.

Karakaş P, Bozkir MG, Oguz O. Morphometric measurements from various reference points in the orbit of male Caucasians. Surg Radiol Anat. 2003;24(6):358–62.

Karim S, Clark RA, Poukens V, Demer JL. Demonstration of systematic variation in human intraorbital optic nerve size by quantitative magnetic resonance imaging and histology. Invest Ophthalmol Vis Sci. 2004;45(4):1047–51.

Kashiwagi K, Okubo T, Tsukahara S. Association of magnetic resonance imaging of anterior optic pathway with glaucomatous visual field damage and optic disc cupping. J Glaucoma. 2004;13(3):189–95.

Laestadius ND, Aase JM, Smith DW. Normal inner canthal and outer orbital dimensions. J Pediatr. 1969;74(3):465–8.

Lee JS, Lim DW, Lee SH, Oum BS, Kim HJ, Lee HJ. Normative measurements of Korean orbital structures revealed by computerized tomography. Acta Ophthalmol Scand. 2001;79(2):197–200.

Lee H, Lee Y, Ha S, Park M, Baek S. Measurement of width and distance of the posterior border of the deep lateral orbital wall using computed tomography. J Craniomaxillofac Surg. 2011;39(8):606–9.

Lee JS, Lee H, Kim JW, Chang M, Park M, Baek S. Computed tomographic dimensions of the lacrimal gland in healthy orbits. J Craniofac Surg. 2013;24(3):712–5.

Lefebvre DR, Yoon MK. CT-based measurements of the sphenoid trigone in different sex and race. Ophthalmic Plast Reconstr Surg. 2015;31(2):155–8.

Lenhart PD, Desai NK, Bruce BB, Hutchinson AK, Lambert SR. The role of magnetic resonance imaging in diagnosing optic nerve hypoplasia. Am J Ophthalmol. 2014;158(6):1164–1171.e2.

Lerdlum S, Boonsirikamchai P, Setsakol E. Normal measurements of extraocular muscle using computed tomography. J Med Assoc Thail. 2007;90(2):307–12.

Lirng JF, Fuh JL, Wu ZA, Lu SR, Wang SJ. Diameter of the superior ophthalmic vein in relation to intracranial pressure. AJNR Am J Neuroradiol. 2003;24(4):700–3.

Mafee MF, Pruzansky S, Corrales MM, Phatak MG, Valvassori GE, Dobben GD, Capek V. CT in the evaluation of the orbit and the bony interorbital distance. AJNR Am J Neuroradiol. 1986;7(2):265–9.

Maresky HS, Ben Ely A, Bartischovsky T, Coret-Simon J, Morad Y, Rozowsky S, Klar M, Negieva S, Bekerman I, Tal S. MRI measurements of the normal pediatric optic nerve pathway. J Clin Neurosci. 2018;48:209–13.

Nam Y, Bahk S, Eo S. Anatomical study of the infraorbital nerve and surrounding structures for the surgery of orbital floor fractures. J Craniofac Surg. 2017;28(4):1099–104.

Nguyen DC, Farber SJ, Um GT, Skolnick GB, Woo AS, Patel KB. Anatomical study of the intraosseous pathway of the infraorbital nerve. J Craniofac Surg. 2016;27(4):1094–7.

Nugent RA, Belkin RI, Neigel JM, Rootman J, Robertson WD, Spinelli J, Graeb DA. Graves orbitopathy: correlation of CT and clinical findings. Radiology. 1990;177(3):675–82.

Ozgen A, Ariyurek M. Normative measurements of orbital structures using CT. AJR Am J Roentgenol. 1998;170(4):1093–6.

Ozgen A, Aydingöz U. Normative measurements of orbital structures using MRI. J Comput Assist Tomogr. 2000;24(3):493–6.

Pool GM, Didier RA, Bardo D, Selden NR, Kuang AA. Computed tomography-generated anthropometric measurements of orbital relationships in normal infants and children. J Neurosurg Pediatr. 2016;18(2):201–6.

Saccà S, Polizzi A, Macrì A, Patrone G, Rolando M. Echographic study of extraocular muscle thickness in children and adults. Eye (Lond). 2000;14(5):765–9.

Shofty B, Ben-Sira L, Constantini S, Freedman S, Kesler A. Optic nerve sheath diameter on MR imaging: establishment of norms and comparison of pediatric patients with idiopathic intracranial hypertension with healthy controls. AJNR Am J Neuroradiol. 2012;33(2):366–9.

Suh JD, Kuan EC, Thompson CF, Scawn RL, Feinstein AJ, Barham HP, Kingdom TT, Ramakrishnan VR. Using fixed anatomical landmarks to avoid medial rectus injury: a radiographic analysis in patients with and without Graves' disease. Am J Otolaryngol. 2016;37(4):334–8.

Swan KC, Wilkins JH. Extraocular muscle surgery in early infancy—anatomical factors. J Pediatr Ophthalmol Strabismus. 1984;21(2):44–9.

Tanitame K, Sone T, Miyoshi T, Tanitame N, Otani K, Akiyama Y, Takasu M, Date S, Kiuchi Y, Awai K. Ocular volumetry using fast high-resolution MRI during visual fixation. AJNR Am J Neuroradiol. 2013;34(4):870–6.

Tian S, Nishida Y, Isberg B, Lennerstrand G. MRI measurements of normal extraocular muscles and other orbital structures. Graefes Arch Clin Exp Ophthalmol. 2000;238(5):393–404.

Tsutsumi S, Nakamura M, Tabuchi T, Yasumoto Y. The superior ophthalmic vein: delineation with high-resolution magnetic resonance imaging. Surg Radiol Anat. 2015;37(1):75–80.

Turvey TA, Golden BA. Orbital anatomy for the surgeon. Oral Maxillofac Surg Clin North Am. 2012;24(4):525–36.

Vaiman M, Abuita R, Bekerman I. Optic nerve sheath diameters in healthy adults measured by computer tomography. Int J Ophthalmol. 2015;8(6):1240–4.

Watcharakorn A, Ngamsirisuk S. Normal measurements of size of optic nerve sheath complex using computed tomography. J Med Assoc Thail. 2014;97(Suppl 8):S22–6.

Weissman JL, Beatty RL, Hirsch WL, Curtin HD. Enlarged anterior chamber: CT finding of a ruptured globe. AJNR Am J Neuroradiol. 1995;16(4 Suppl):936–8.

Normative Measurements of Temporal Bone Structures on Imaging

3

Daniel Thomas Ginat and Michael B. Gluth

3.1 External Auditory Canal

- The external auditory canal is a slightly curved passage from the auricle to the tympanic membrane.
- The lateral 1/3 is comprised of cartilage, while the medial 2/3 is comprised of bone.
- In adults, the external auditory canal is approximately 22–25 mm long from the concha of the auricle to the tympanic membrane (Fig. 3.1).
- The average height of the external auditory canal is 9–10 mm and the average width is 6–7 mm (Fig. 3.2).
- The tympanic membrane terminates the external auditory canal at an angle of 45–60° with an obtuse angle at the posterior aspect of the tympanic membrane and an acute angle at the anterior tympanomeatal sulcus. Consequently, the posterior

D. T. Ginat (✉)
Department of Radiology, Section of Neuroradiology,
University of Chicago, Chicago, IL, USA
e-mail: dtg1@uchicago.edu

M. B. Gluth
Department of Surgery, Section of Otolaryngology-Head and Neck Surgery, University of Chicago, Chicago, IL, USA

© Springer Nature Switzerland AG 2021
D. T. Ginat (ed.), *Manual of Normative Measurements in Head and Neck Imaging*, https://doi.org/10.1007/978-3-030-50567-7_3

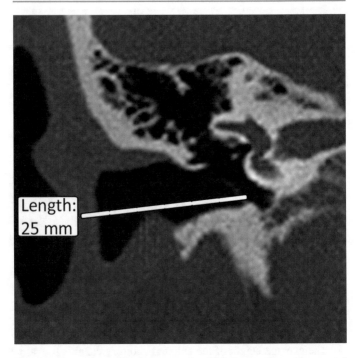

Fig. 3.1 Coronal computed tomography (CT) image shows the normal length of the external auditory canal

ear canal is approximately 6 mm shorter along the posterior wall as compared to the anterior wall.
- The anterior canal wall can have a bulge of a few millimeters into the lumen of the external auditory canal according to the contour of the underlying temporomandibular joint capsule.

Practical Implications
- The external auditory canal can be narrow with congenital aural atresia and can have a residual stenotic lumen or can be completely filled with soft tissue (Fig. 3.3).
- A widening external auditory canal can result from canaloplasty (Fig. 3.4).

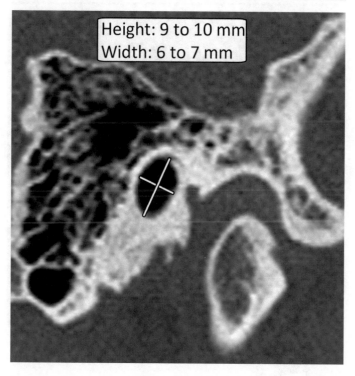

Height: 9 to 10 mm
Width: 6 to 7 mm

Fig. 3.2 Sagittal computed tomography (CT) image shows the normal diameter of the external auditory canal

3.2   Middle Ear Cavity

- The middle ear cavity is an air-filled cavity within the petrous portion of the temporal bone that contains the ossicular chain and is bounded by the tympanic membrane laterally, the cochlear promontory medially, the tegmen tympani superiorly, the mastoid wall posteriorly, and the jugular wall and hypotympanic air cells inferiorly.
- The average volume of the middle ear is 5.2 ± 3.1 mm^3 (range: 0.6–13.4 mm^3).

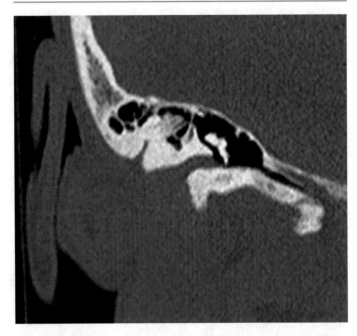

Fig. 3.3 Coronal computed tomography (CT) image shows a narrow bony external auditory canal, which is filled with soft tissue in a patient with external auditory atresia

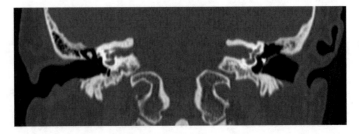

Fig. 3.4 Coronal computed tomography (CT) image shows a widened left external auditory canal from canaloplasty for ossicular reconstruction

- The middle ear cavity is divided into the following compartments:
  - Mesotympanum immediately deep to the tympanic membrane
  - Epitympanum superior and deep to the pars flaccida and scutum wherein the ossicular heads and chorda tympani are located
  - Retrotympanum posterior and deep to the tympanic ring wherein the pyramidal process and sinus tympani are located
  - Protympanum anterior and deep to tympanic ring wherein carotid canal and Eustachian tube orifice are located
  - Hypotympanum inferior and deep to the tympanic ring wherein the jugular bulb and infracochlear hypotympanic air cells are located.
- There is variable pneumatization of the space between the facial nerve and the chorda tympani known as the facial recess, but often this space is a surgical potential space predominately filled with bone. The facial recess is triangular in shape and widest superiorly where it is 2–3 mm in greatest width. The facial recess is a common route of surgical dissection into the middle ear space via mastoidectomy approaches.
- Potentially important areas in the middle ear that are especially relevant during surgical dissection of cholesteatoma include the following:
  - The anterior epitympanic recess (supratubal recess) is a space continuous with the anterior epitympanum. It is located anterior to the malleus head and cog (an embryologic remnant bony crest that separates the posterior epitympanum from the anterior epitympanum that arises as a projection from the tegmen tympani). It is also located superior to the tensor tympani muscle and canal. The supratubal recess is usually a single air cell, but there are variants where the space is comprised of multiple cells. It measures 3 mm in width with a range of 1–7 mm (Fig. 3.5).

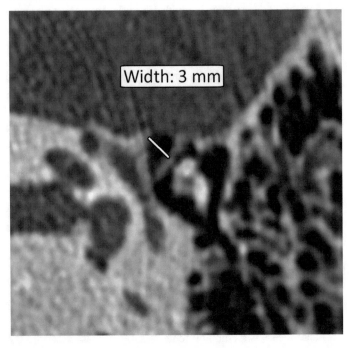

Fig. 3.5 Axial computed tomography (CT) image shows the width of a normal epitympanic recess located anterior to the cog

- The retrotympanum includes the facial recess and the sinus tympani medial to the proximal segment of the facial nerve. The sinus tympani has been classified into differing subtypes depending on its depth relative to the adjacent facial nerve:

    Type A is shallow with limited extension medial to the nerve.

    Type B (most common) extends medial to the entire facial nerve width.

    Type C extends posteriorly beyond the width of the facial nerve, often communicating with the mastoid air cells (Fig. 3.6).

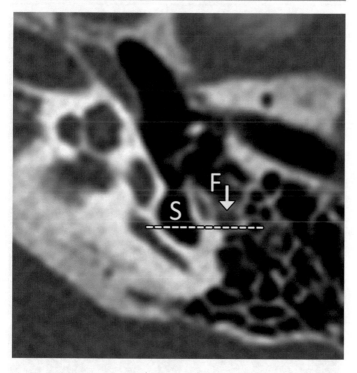

Fig. 3.6 Axial computed tomography (CT) image shows a deep (Type C) sinus tympani (S) extending posterior to the mastoid segment of the facial nerve (arrow). A pneumatized facial nerve recess (F) is present lateral to the facial nerve

Practical Implications

- The middle ear can be underdeveloped with diminished volume in association with otitis media during childhood or in association with congenital aural atresia (Fig. 3.7). There are acoustic implications for a small volume tympanic cleft insofar as the degree of hearing loss associated with a given tympanic membrane perforation will be more severe if the middle ear volume is excessively low.

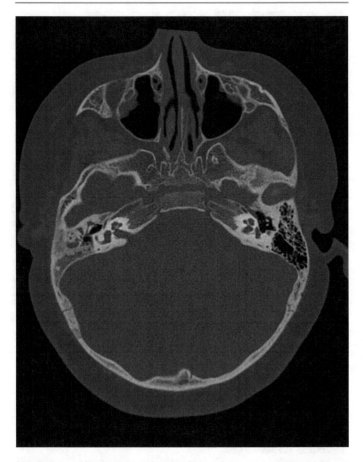

Fig. 3.7 Axial computed tomography (CT) image shows a relatively small right middle ear cavity, along with deficiency of the ossicles and underpneumatized mastoid air cells in a patient with external auditory canal atresia

- Sinus tympani depth can influence surgical preference in cholesteatoma surgery. For example, with a shallow recess, an exclusive transcanal approach can be adequate; while with a deep (Type C) recess can warrant a transmastoid retrofacial approach.
- The anterior epitympanic recess is a noteworthy site for involvement with cholesteatoma that is difficult to clear surgically.

3.3   Tympanic Membrane

- The normal tympanic membrane has submillimeter thickness (average of 70 μm) and a shallow cone-like shape, which is normally only faintly discernible on CT (Fig. 3.8).
- It has a diameter of 8–10 mm and a surface area of 55–90 mm^2 with a mean value of 65 mm^2.
- The tympanic membrane has two components, the pars tensa and the pars flaccida.
- The peripheral margins of pars tensa originate from the fibrous annulus, which is near-circumferentially embedded in a groove of the tympanic bone known as the tympanic ring. The radial collagenous fibers of the pars tensa are slightly bowed and extend to the central attachment of the pars tensa to the malleus

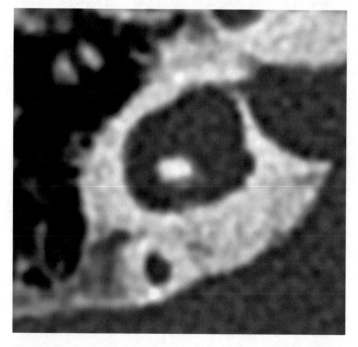

Fig. 3.8   Axial computed tomography (CT) image shows the thin, faintly visible normal tympanic membrane (arrows)

manubrium, which is situated is 1–2 mm medial to the orientation of the tympanic ring. The malleus attachment extends from the central umbo to the superior lateral process.

- The pars flaccida (Shrapnells membrane) is a small triangular segment of tympanic membrane that is superior to the malleus short process and lateral to the malleus neck. It extends over the tympanic notch (notch of Rivinus) and it has an average surface area of 3 mm^2.

Practical Implications
- The pars flaccida is the most common site of acquired cholesteatoma development, and thickening or soft tissue underlying this area should be viewed with suspicion (Fig. 3.9).
- If the pars tensa can be prominently viewed on CT scan, this may suggest pathologic thickening, such as myringosclerosis, or postsurgical changes (Figs. 3.10 and 3.11).

3.4   Ossicular Chain

Malleus: The malleus is comprised of a head, neck, anterior process, lateral process, and manubrium.

- The malleus has the following average dimensions (Fig. 3.12):
  - Total length: 7.8 mm
  - Length of manubrium: 4.7 mm
  - Length of head and neck of malleus: 4.9 mm
- The mean distance between the cochlear promontory and the handle of the malleus is 1.7 mm; however, the malleus pivots around a fulcrum generated at the anterior process near the malleus neck and the anteriorly projecting anterior malleal ligament, which attaches to the anterior/superior tympanic ring. Due to this potential rotation, the distance between the umbo of the manubrium and promontory can vary over time depending on the pressure equalization status of the middle ear (Fig. 3.13).

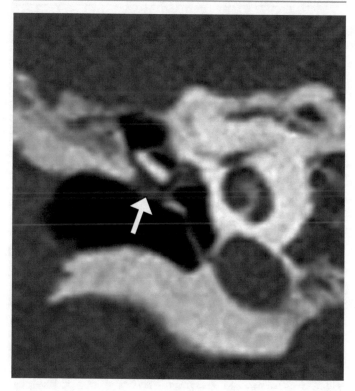

Fig. 3.9 Coronal computed tomography (CT) image shows opacification of the Prussak space due to a pars flaccida cholesteatoma (arrow), with truncation of the scutum

Incus: The incus is comprised of a body, short process, long process and lenticular process. The incus has the following average dimensions (Fig. 3.14):

- Total length: 5.4 mm
- Maximum width: 2.5 mm
- Long process diameter: 0.6 mm

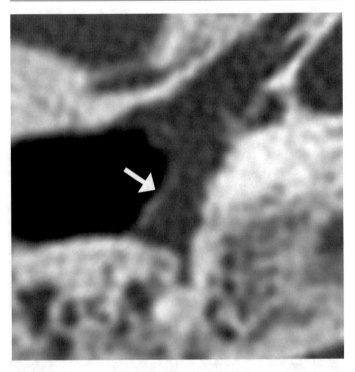

Fig. 3.10 Axial computed tomography (CT) image shows thickening and calcification of the tympanic membrane (arrow) due to myringosclerosis. There is also opacification of the middle ear cavity

Stapes: The stapes is comprised of a capitulum, anterior and posterior crus, and a footplate that attaches to the oval window. The stapes has the following average dimensions (Fig. 3.15):

- The mean height of the stapes is 3.3 mm (95% confidence interval: 3.3–3.4 mm)
- The mean length of the footplates is 2.7 mm (95% confidence interval: 2.7–2.8 mm)
- The mean width of the footplates is 1.1 mm (95% confidence interval: 0.9–1.3)

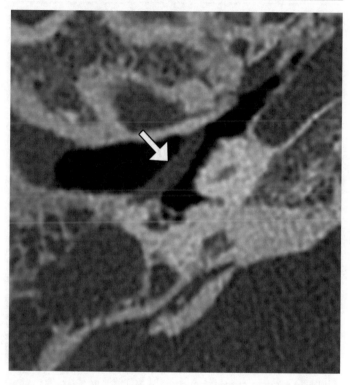

Fig. 3.11 Axial computed tomography (CT) shows a cartilage tympanoplasty graft (arrow)

- The stapes axial plane is directed upward, outward (44°), and forward (12°) with respect to the lateral semicircular canal plane.
- The posterior crus is usually slightly thicker than the anterior crus.
- The dimensions of the stapes tend to be bilaterally symmetrical.
- The mean incudostapedial angle is 82°, with a range of 66–96° (Fig. 3.16).

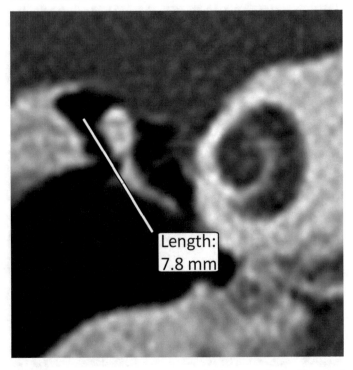

Fig. 3.12 Coronal computed tomography (CT) image shows the normal length of the malleus

Practical Implications

- The ossicles can be shortened due to developmental malformations, inflammatory conditions, and tumors (Fig. 3.17).
- The thickness of the stapes footplate can be considered enlarged when measuring at least 0.7 mm on axial sections, which can result from otosclerosis, chronic otitis media, and malformations (Fig. 3.18).
- There can be increased distance from the cochlear promontory to the handle of the malleus in patients with congenital ossicular abnormalities.

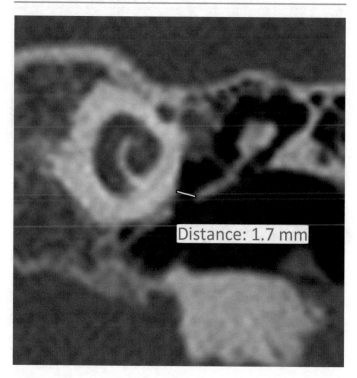

Fig. 3.13 Coronal computed tomography (CT) image shows the normal distance between the mandibular handle and cochlear promontory

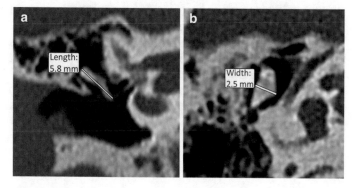

Fig. 3.14 Coronal (**a**) and axial (**b**) computed tomography (CT) images show the normal length and width of the incus

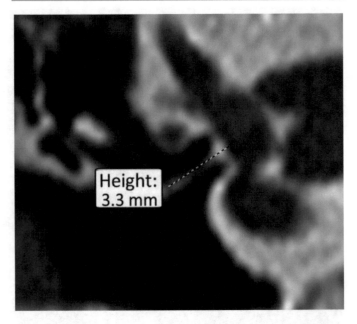

Fig. 3.15 Coronal computed tomography (CT) image shows the length of a normal stapes

3.5 Mastoid Air Cells

- The mastoid bone is normally pneumatized with a complex of interconnected air cells (Fig. 3.19).
- The antrum is developed at birth and in parallel with the pneumatization; the mastoid bone expansion rate is about 0.6–0.9 cm/year in length and width and 0.4 cm/year in depth in the first year, followed by half that rate until up to 7 years, with a slower growth rate during puberty until reaching adult size.

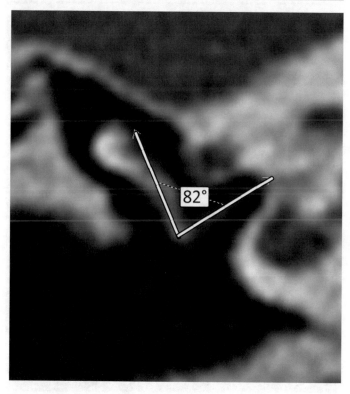

Fig. 3.16 Coronal computed tomography (CT) image shows the normal incudostapedial angle

- The mean volume of the mastoid air cell pneumatization in adults is about 8 cm³, with a range of 4.0–14.0 cm³.
- There is a plate of bone dividing the squamous portion (superficial) of the mastoid from the petrous portion (deep) of the mastoid known as the Koerner septum. The degree of pneumatization of each of these portions of the mastoid relative to one another may vary in some normal cases.

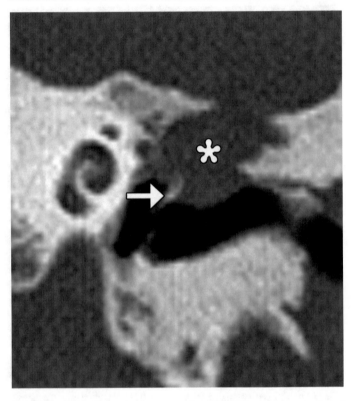

Fig. 3.17 Coronal computed tomography (CT) image shows a truncated malleus (arrow) due to erosion by a cholesteatoma (*)

Practical Implications
- Restricted temporal bone pneumatization is a possible consequence of tympanomastoid dysventilation and/or infection during childhood development.
- An isolated grouping of opacified air cells in the mastoid tip region and the adjacent inferior portion of the retrosig-

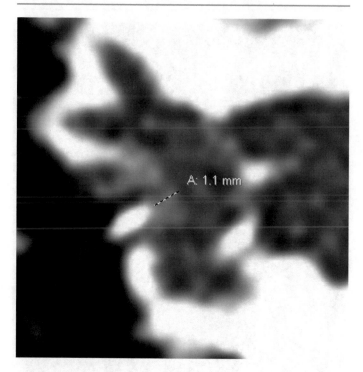

Fig. 3.18 Coronal computed tomography (CT) image shows thickening of the footplate and abnormal surrounding bone in a patient with otosclerosis treated with a stapes prosthesis

moid air cell tract may be a normal variant from bone marrow.
- Sclerotic patterns of temporal bone pneumatization are often associated with chronic otitis media and possibly cholesteatoma—especially involving the epitympanum (Fig. 3.20).

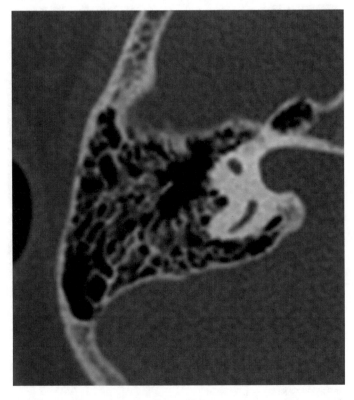

Fig. 3.19 Axial computed tomography (CT) image shows normal pneumatization of the right mastoid air cells in a child

3.6   Facial Nerve Canal

- The intratemporal facial nerve consists of the labyrinthine, tympanic, and mastoid segments.
- There is slight progressive widening of the facial nerve canal through the temporal bone distally (Fig. 3.21).
- In roughly 70% of normal subjects, the distal segment of the mastoid segment travels in a trajectory that courses lateral to

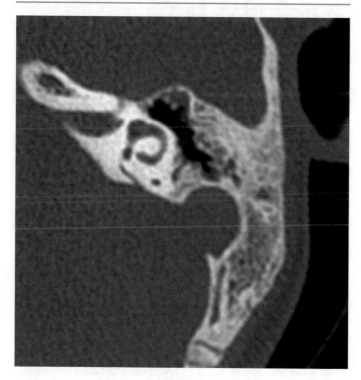

Fig. 3.20 Axial computed tomography (CT) image shows significantly restricted pneumatization of the squamous portion of the left mastoid, while still having some degree of petrous mastoid air cell formation around the antrum in a child with prior otitis media

   the plane of the inferior aspect of the tympanic annulus in close proximity to the posterior inferior aspect of the bony external auditory canal.
- The most common segment of the facial nerve to be dehiscent is the tympanic segment and this is radiologically present on CT in 20–30% of normal cases.

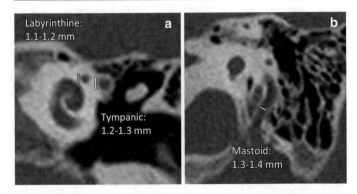

Fig. 3.21 Coronal computed tomography (CT) images (**a** and **b**) show the typical diameters of the labyrinthine, tympanic, and mastoid segments of the facial nerve. Note the progressive widening

- The normal average short axis diameter of nerve canals is as follows:
  - Labyrinthine segment: 1.1–1.2 mm, standard deviation: 0.3 mm
  - Tympanic segment: 1.2–1.3 mm, standard deviation: 0.2 mm
  - Mastoid segment: 1.3–1.4 mm, standard deviation: 0.2 mm

- The upper limits of the 95% confidence intervals for left–right asymmetry are 0.25, 0.21, and 0.15 mm for the labyrinthine, tympanic, and mastoid segments of the facial nerve canal, respectively.

Practical Implications
- Symmetry of the canal size is more indicative of normal than the actual diameter and enlargement can be caused by tumors, such as schwannomas (Fig. 3.22).
- The dehiscent facial nerve is a common finding in the tympanic segment, which can put it at risk of injury during middle ear surgery.
- The distal aspect of the mastoid segment of the facial nerve is often at risk of injury during surgery of the posterior–inferior external auditory canal due to its orientation lateral to the tympanic annulus.

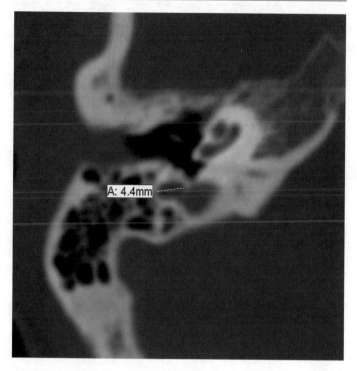

Fig. 3.22 Axial CT image shows widening of the mastoid segment of the right facial nerve canal due to a tumor

3.7   Cochlea

- The cochlea is a spiral-shaped inner ear structure within the petrous temporal bone with approximately 2.5 turns.
- The cochlea is completely developed and reaches adult size at birth.
- The mean dimensions of the cochlea are as follows (Fig. 3.23):
  - Cochlear length: 9.1 mm
  - Cochlear height: 5.1 mm
  - Basal Turn Lumen Diameter: 1.5–2.7 mm
- Cochlear height does not change from 1 month of age to adulthood and is slightly greater in males than in females

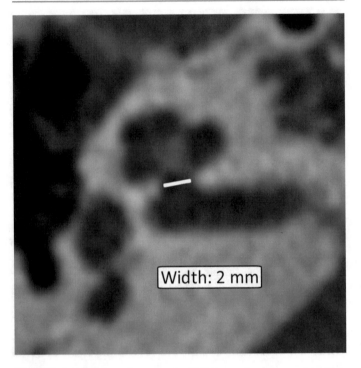

Width: 2 mm

Fig. 3.23 Axial computed tomography (CT) image shows a normal cochlear aperture diameter

- Round window with the following dimensions (Fig. 3.24):
  - Diameter: 2.0 mm
  - Area: 2.1–2.3 mm²
- The cochlear nerve canal (cochlear aperture, bony cochlear nerve canal, or cochlear fossette) is a passage for the cochlear nerve between the internal auditory canal and the modiolus.
- The mean cochlear nerve canal diameter is approximately 2 mm (Fig. 3.25).
- The cochlear aperture can be considered abnormally narrow if it measures less than 1.4 mm in width and abnormally wide if it measures greater than 3.0 mm in width on axial images.

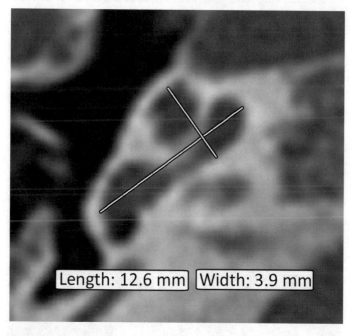

Fig. 3.24 Axial computed tomography (CT) image shows the average dimensions of the cochlea

- The cochlear aqueduct is a funnel-shaped channel through the petrous bone that contains the perilymphatic duct from the scala tympani to the subarachnoid space and has the following mean dimensions (Fig. 3.26):
  - Cochlear aqueduct length: 12.6 mm
  - Cochlear aqueduct medial width: 3.9 mm

Practical Implications
- Stenosis of the cochlear aperture is associated with sensorineural hearing loss due to cochlear nerve deficiency, which is best depicted on magnetic resonance imaging (MRI) (Fig. 3.27).

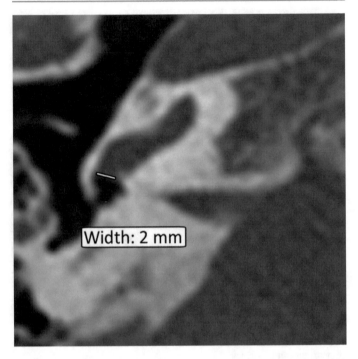

Fig. 3.25 Axial computed tomography (CT) image shows the average width of the round window

- Cochlear hypoplasia with a height of less than 4.4 mm has a positive predictive value of 100% for sensorineural hearing loss (Fig. 3.28).
- Variability in the size of the cochlea can have implications in choosing the optimal length of a cochlear implant electrode.
- The length of the cochlear electrodes for a 270° insertion depth can be determined from the diameter of the basal turn of the cochlea (D) depicted on a minimum intensity projection CT image shown in Fig. 3.29 using the following equation:

$$\text{Cochlear implant length} = 2.62 \times D \times \log\left(1 + 270/235\right)$$

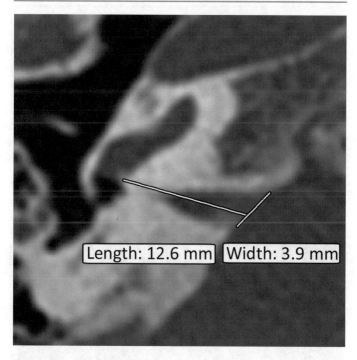

Fig. 3.26 Axial computed tomography (CT) image shows the average dimensions of the cochlear aqueduct

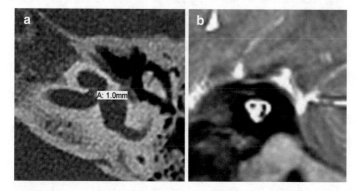

Fig. 3.27 Axial computed tomography (CT) image (**a**) shows a narrow cochlear aperture (**b**). The sagittal oblique T2-weighted MRI shows deficiency of the cochlear nerve

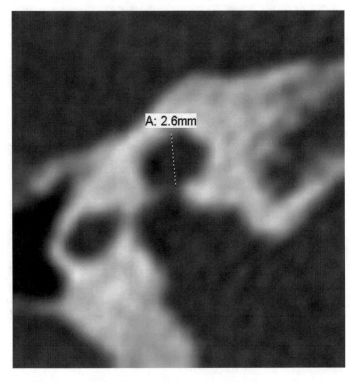

Fig. 3.28 Axial computed tomography (CT) image shows a hypoplastic cochlea in a patient with branchio-oto-renal syndrome

3.8 Vestibule

- The vestibule is an ovoid space located superior and posterior to the cochlea, which connects to the semicircular canals.
- The dimensions of the vestibule in the axial plane are as follows (Fig. 3.30):
  - Length: 5.9 ± 0.3, range: 5.2–6.6 mm
  - Width: 2.5 ± 0.4, range 1.8–3.2 mm
  - Area: 14.0 ± 1.7, range 10.6–17.3 mm^2

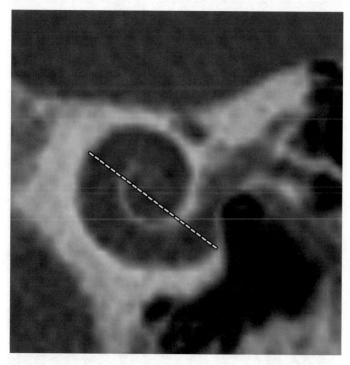

Fig. 3.29 Minimum intensity projection computed tomography (CT) image shows the diameter of the cochlear basal turn (dashed line) for determining cochlear implant insertion length

- The dimensions of the vestibule in the coronal plane are as follows (Fig. 3.31):
  - Length: 5.1 ± 0.3, range: 4.4–5.7 mm
  - Width: 2.4 ± 0.2, range: 2.0–2.8 mm
  - Area: 11.3 ± 1.3, range: 8.7–13.9 mm^2
- The oval window is an opening in the lateral aspect of the vestibule. While the oval window actually has an oval shape in 53% of cases, it can have other shapes, such as kidney, D shape, rectangular, and trapezoidal configurations.

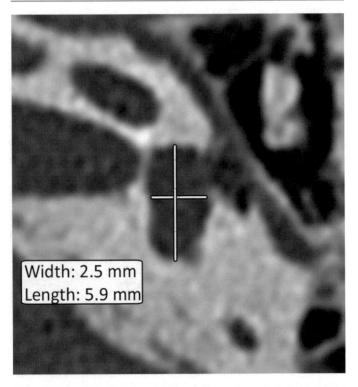

Width: 2.5 mm
Length: 5.9 mm

Fig. 3.30 Axial computed tomography (CT) image shows the dimensions of a normal vestibule

- The mean height and width of the oval window are 1.3 ± 0.3 mm and 2.7 ± 0.4 mm, respectively (Fig. 3.32).

Practical Implications
- Oval window atresia can be associated with facial nerve and stapes anomalies, as well as a small middle ear cavity (Fig. 3.33).
- Measurement of the oval window height is relevant to otosclerosis surgery. A narrow window should be considered at risk for technical difficulties during the stapes footplate approach.

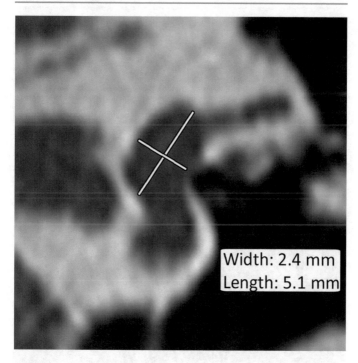

Fig. 3.31 Coronal computed tomography (CT) image shows the dimensions of a normal vestibule

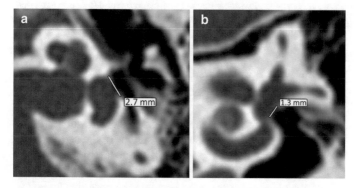

Fig. 3.32 Axial (**a**) and coronal (**b**) computed tomography (CT) images show the dimensions of a normal oval window

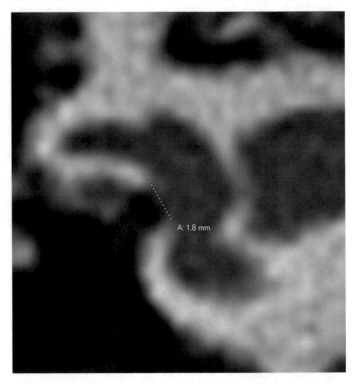

Fig. 3.33 Oval window atresia. Coronal computed tomography (CT) image shows a narrow oval window (arrow) and markedly underpneumatized middle ear in the setting of external auditory atresia, with absence of the stapes and displaced facial nerve canal

3.9   Vestibular Aqueduct

- The vestibular aqueduct arises from the medial wall of the vestibule and extends to the posterior surface of the petrous bone.
- The distal portion of the vestibular aqueduct turns inferiorly and has a triangular configuration with the apex at the isthmus and the base (aperture) projecting into the posterior fossa.

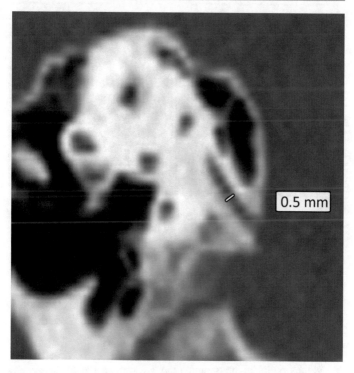

Fig. 3.34 Sagittal oblique computed tomography (CT) image shows the normal width of the vestibular aqueduct in cross-section

- In the 45° sagittal oblique plane, the vestibular aqueduct is depicted in cross-section with a normal mean midpoint width of 0.5 mm that ranges from 0.3 to 0.9 mm (Fig. 3.34).
- In the axial plane, according to the Valvassori criterion, the vestibular aqueduct is considered enlarged if it measures at least 1.5 mm at the midpoint, while the Cincinnati criteria consider the vestibular aqueduct enlarged if it measures more than 0.9 mm at the midpoint or more than 1.9 mm at the operculum (Fig. 3.35).

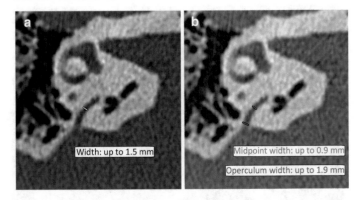

Fig. 3.35 Axial computed tomography (CT) images show the upper limits of size of the vestibular aqueduct based on the Valvassori criterion (**a**) and the Cincinnati criteria (**b**)

- The midpoint width on axial images is measured at the bisection of a line from the posterior wall of the vestibular aqueduct, perpendicular to the ray measuring the operculum width.

Practical Implications

- Values equal to or greater than 1.2 mm in the midpoint and 1.3 mm in the operculum are proposed criteria to diagnose enlarged vestibular aqueduct in the 45° oblique reformatted images (Fig. 3.36).
- The Cincinnati criterion is more sensitive than Valvassori criteria in the diagnosis of enlarged vestibular aqueduct syndrome.
- Enlarged vestibular aqueduct measures twice the width of the adjacent posterior semicircular canal.

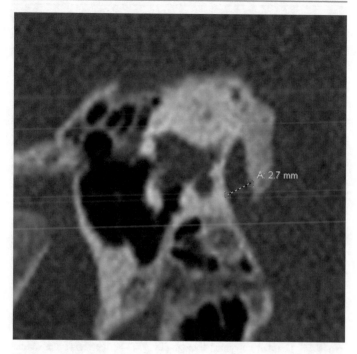

Fig. 3.36 Sagittal oblique computed tomography (CT) image shows enlargement of the vestibular aqueduct in a patient with incomplete partition type 2

3.10   Semicircular Canals

- The semicircular canals detect angular accelerations and are comprised of the orthogonally oriented lateral (horizontal), superior (vertical), and posterior semicircular canals, in which the superior and posterior share a common crus.
- The semicircular canals are slightly ovoid in cross-section, with normal average diameters distal to the ampulae of 1.2 by 1.4 mm (Fig. 3.37).

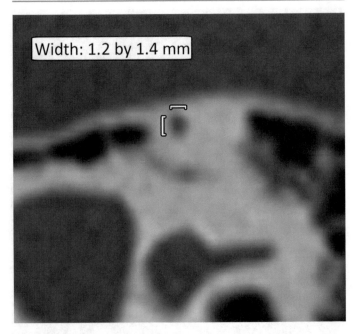

Fig. 3.37 Coronal computed tomography (CT) image shows the normal cross-sectional dimensions of the semicircular canal

- The thickness of bone overlying the superior semicircular canal in the coronal plane in 90% of normal patients is at least 0.4 mm, with an average of 1.3 mm (Fig. 3.38).
- The normal average lateral semicircular canal bony island width is 3.7 mm (range: 2.6–4.8 mm) (Fig. 3.39).

Practical Implications
- Deficiency of the bone over the superior semicircular canal can lead to dehiscence (Fig. 3.40).
- Lateral semicircular canal dysplasia with a small bone island can be isolated or a manifestation of Down syndrome and can be associated with hyperacusis (Fig. 3.41).

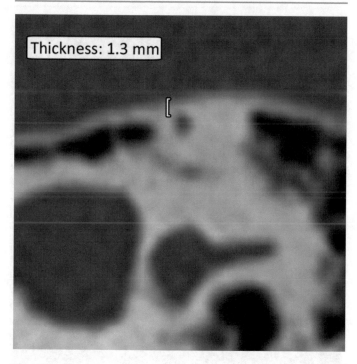

Fig. 3.38 Coronal computed tomography (CT) image shows the normal thickness of bone overlying the superior semicircular canal

3.11   Internal Auditory Canal

- The internal auditory canal extends from the posteromedial surface of the petrous pyramid to the cribriform plate, which closes the canal laterally and separates the canal from the vestibule.
- The canal transmits the cochlear and vestibular divisions, the facial nerve, the nervus intermedius, and the labyrinthine artery.
- The diameter of the normal internal auditory canal varies from 2 mm to 12 mm, with an average diameter of 5–6 mm, and measures 15–20 mm in length (Fig. 3.42).

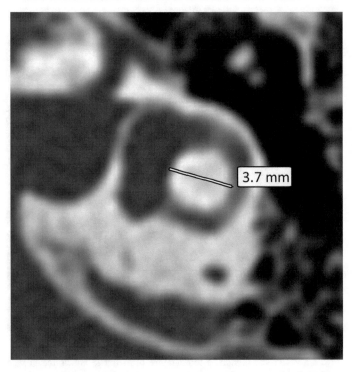

Fig. 3.39 Axial computed tomography (CT) image shows a normal bone island

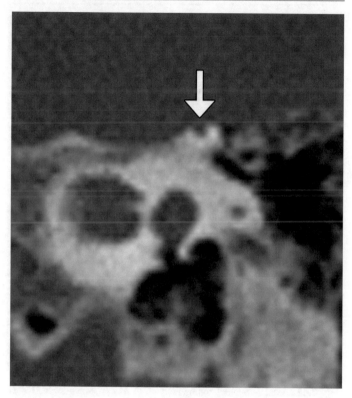

Fig. 3.40 Stenver reformat computed tomography (CT) image shows superior semicircular canal dehiscence (arrow)

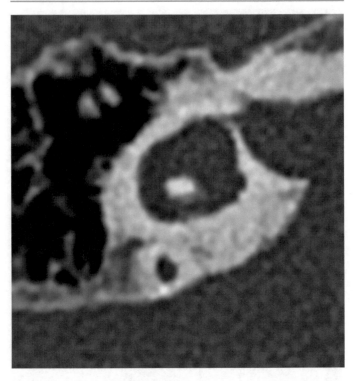

Fig. 3.41 Axial computed tomography (CT) image shows a small bone island with dilatation of both the anterior and posterior arms of the lateral semicircular canal

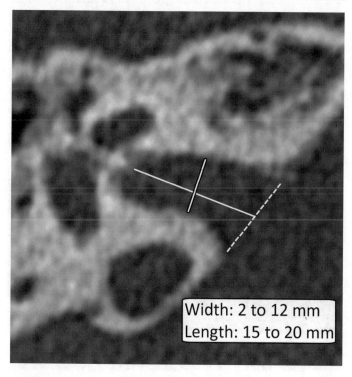

Width: 2 to 12 mm
Length: 15 to 20 mm

Fig. 3.42 Axial computed tomography (CT) image denotes the normal dimensions of the internal auditory canal (the dashed line delineates the porous acusticus)

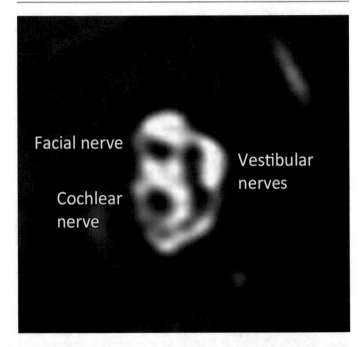

Fig. 3.43 Sagittal oblique T2-weighted magnetic resonance imaging (MRI) shows cranial nerves in the internal auditory canal. The cochlear nerve is thicker than the facial nerve. Note that these nerves are ovoid in cross-section. The superior and inferior vestibular nerves are inseparable

- Although the internal auditory canals in different individuals can differ greatly in size, the two canals of any person are identical or vary by no more than 1 mm.
- The cranial nerves in the internal auditory canals are best delineated on high-resolution T2-weighted sagittal oblique MRI sequences (Fig. 3.43).
- The cochlear nerve is normally larger in cross section than the facial nerve with a maximum diameter of 1.1 versus 1.0 mm.
- The superior and inferior vestibular nerve branches are often inseparable on cross-sectional imaging.

Practical Implications

- Expansion of the internal auditory canal can result from, dural ectasia in neurofibromatosis type II, X-Linked Deafness with Stapes Gusher, and tumors (Fig. 3.44).
- A diverticulum of the anterior–inferior aspect of the internal auditory canal can be a normal variant, but it is associated with possible sensorineural hearing loss of uncertain origin or otosclerosis.
- Congenital narrowing of the internal auditory canal can be associated with deficiency of the vestibulocochlear nerve (Fig. 3.45).
- Acquired stenosis of the canal can be caused by osteomas, meningiomas, fibrous dysplasia, Paget disease, osteopetrosis, Engelmann's disease, and other more unusual bony dysplasias.

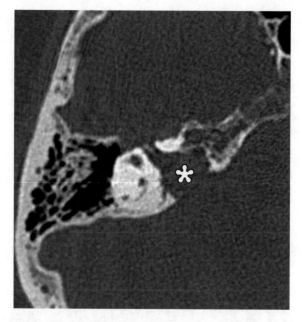

Fig. 3.44 Axial CT image shows widening and irregularity of the right internal auditory canal due to tumor

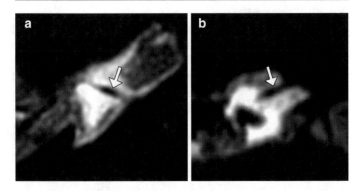

Fig. 3.45 Axial (**a**) and coronal (**b**) computed tomography (CT) images show a narrow internal auditory canal (arrows) that only transmits the facial nerve in a patient with common cavity malformation

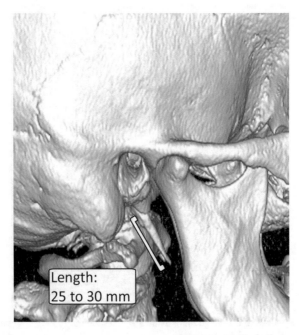

Fig. 3.46 3D computed tomography (CT) image shows a normal styloid process

Styloid Process

- The styloid process is a bony projection from the inferior aspect of the temporal bone and serves to anchor several muscles.
- The normal average length of the styloid process is 25–30 mm with a range between 15 and 48 mm (Fig. 3.46).

Practical implications: An elongated styloid process can lead to cervical pain and dysphagia as part of Eagle syndrome (Fig. 3.47).

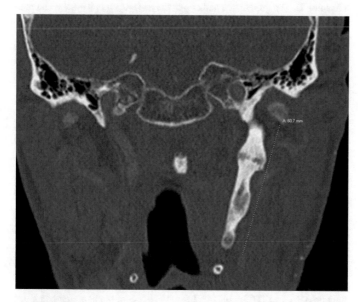

Fig. 3.47 Coronal computed tomography (CT) image shows a markedly elongated and thickened left styloid process in a patient with Eagle syndrome

Further Reading

Ahn JY, Park HJ, Park GH, Jeong YS, Kwak HB, Lee YJ, Shin JE, Moon WJ. Tympanometry and CT measurement of middle ear volumes in patients with unilateral chronic otitis media. Clin Exp Otorhinolaryngol. 2008;1(3):139–42.

Alicandri-Ciufelli M, Fermi M, Bonali M, et al. Facial sinus endoscopic evaluation, radiologic assessment, and classification. Laryngoscope. 2018;128(10):2397–402.

Badhey A, Jategaonkar A, Anglin Kovacs AJ, et al. Eagle syndrome: a comprehensive review. Clin Neurol Neurosurg. 2017;159:34–8.

Calligas JP, Todd NW Jr. Microcomputed tomography of the stapes: wide-ranging dimensions. Ear Nose Throat J. 2018;97(4–5):116–21.

Cinamon U. The growth rate and size of the mastoid air cell system and mastoid bone: a review and reference. Eur Arch Otorhinolaryngol. 2009;266(6):781–6.

El-Badry MM, Osman NM, Mohamed HM, Rafaat FM. Evaluation of the radiological criteria to diagnose large vestibular aqueduct syndrome. Int J Pediatr Otorhinolaryngol. 2016;81:84–91.

Erkoç MF, Imamoglu H, Okur A, Gümüş C, Dogan M. Normative size evaluation of internal auditory canal with magnetic resonance imaging: review of 3786 patients. Folia Morphol (Warsz). 2012;71(4):217–20.

Fatterpekar GM, Mukherji SK, Lin Y, Alley JG, Stone JA, Castillo M. Normal canals at the fundus of the internal auditory canal: CT evaluation. J Comput Assist Tomogr. 1999;23(5):776–80.

Jacob R, Gupta S, Isaacson B, Kutz JW Jr, Roland P, Xi Y, Booth TN. High-resolution CT findings in children with a normal pinna or grade I microtia and unilateral mild stenosis of the external auditory canal. AJNR Am J Neuroradiol. 2015;36(1):176–80.

Jaryszak EM, Patel NA, Camp M, Mancuso AA, Antonelli PJ. Cochlear nerve diameter in normal hearing ears using high-resolution magnetic resonance imaging. Laryngoscope. 2009;119(10):2042–5.

Juliano AF, Ginat DT, Moonis G. Imaging review of the temporal bone: part I. Anatomy and inflammatory and neoplastic processes. Radiology. 2013;269(1):17–33.

Juliano AF, Ginat DT, Moonis G. Imaging review of the temporal bone: part II. Traumatic, postoperative, and noninflammatory nonneoplastic conditions. Radiology. 2015;276(3):655–72.

Juliano AF, Ting EY, Mingkwansook V, Hamberg LM, Curtin HD. Vestibular aqueduct measurements in the 45° oblique (Pöschl) plane. AJNR Am J Neuroradiol. 2016;37(7):1331–7.

Kang WS, Hyun SM, Lim HK, Shim BS, Cho JH, Lee KS. Normative diameters and effects of aging on the cochlear and facial nerves in normal-hearing Korean ears using 3.0-tesla magnetic resonance imaging. Laryngoscope. 2012;122(5):1109–14.

Koç A, Ekinci G, Bilgili AM, Akpinar IN, Yakut H, Han T. Evaluation of the mastoid air cell system by high resolution computed tomography: three-dimensional multiplanar volume rendering technique. J Laryngol Otol. 2003;117(8):595–8.

Kono T. Computed tomographic features of the bony canal of the cochlear nerve in pediatric patients with unilateral sensorineural hearing loss. Radiat Med. 2008;26(3):115–9.

Krombach GA, van den Boom M, Di Martino E, et al. Computed tomography of the inner ear: size of anatomical structures in the normal temporal bone and in the temporal bone of patients with Menière's disease. Eur Radiol. 2005;15(8):1505–13.

Lee DH, Jun BC, Kim DG, Jung MK, Yeo SW. Volume variation of mastoid pneumatization in different age groups: a study by three-dimensional reconstruction based on computed tomography images. Surg Radiol Anat. 2005;27(1):37–42.

Lou J, Gong WX, Wang GB. Cochlear nerve diameters on multipoint measurements and effects of aging in normal-hearing children using 3.0-T magnetic resonance imaging. Int J Pediatr Otorhinolaryngol. 2015;79(7):1077–80.

Marchioni D, Valerini S, Mattioli F, Alicandri-Ciufelli M, Presutti L. Radiological assessment of the sinus tympani: temporal bone HRCT analyses and surgically related findings. Surg Radiol Anat. 2015;37(4):385–92.

Miyasaka M, Nosaka S, Morimoto N, Taiji H, Masaki H. CT and MR imaging for pediatric cochlear implantation: emphasis on the relationship between the cochlear nerve canal and the cochlear nerve. Pediatr Radiol. 2010;40(9):1509–16.

Mori MC, Chang KW. CT analysis demonstrates that cochlear height does not change with age. AJNR Am J Neuroradiol. 2012;33(1):119–23.

Noussios G, Chouridis P, Kostretzis L, Natsis K. Morphological and morphometrical study of the human ossicular Chain: a review of the literature and a meta-analysis of experience over 50 years. J Clin Med Res. 2016;8(2):76–83.

Park JH, Kang SI, Choi HS, Lee SY, Kim JS, Koo JW. Thickness of the bony otic capsule: etiopathogenetic perspectives on superior canal dehiscence syndrome. Audiol Neurootol. 2015;20(4):243–50.

Pelliccia P, Venail F, Bonafé A, et al. Cochlea size variability and implications in clinical practice. Acta Otorhinolaryngol Ital. 2014;34(1):42–9.

Petrus LV, Lo WW. The anterior epitympanic recess: CT anatomy and pathology. AJNR Am J Neuroradiol. 1997;18(6):1109–14.

Pippin KJ, Muelleman TJ, Hill J, Leever J, Staecker H, Ledbetter LN. Prevalence of internal auditory canal diverticulum and its association with hearing loss and otosclerosis. Am J Neuroradiol. 2017;38(11):2167–71.

Prasad KC, Kamath MP, Reddy KJ, Raju K, Agarwal S. Elongated styloid process (Eagle's Syndrome): a clinical study. J Oral Maxillofac Surg. 2002;60:171–5.

Purcell DD, Fischbein NJ, Patel A, Johnson J, Lalwani AK. Two temporal bone computed tomography measurements increase recognition of malformations and predict sensorineural hearing loss. Laryngoscope. 2006;116(8):1439–46.

Rask-Andersen H, Liu W, Erixon E, Kinnefors A, Pfaller K, Schrott-Fischer A, Glueckert R. Human cochlea: anatomical characteristics and their relevance for cochlear implantation. Anat Rec (Hoboken). 2012;295(11):1791–811.

Rousset J, Garetier M, Gentric JC, Chinellato S, Barberot C, Le Bivic T, Mériot P. Biometry of the normal stapes using stapes axial plane, high-resolution computed tomography. J Laryngol Otol. 2014;128(5):425–30.

Sepahdari AR, Mong S. Skull base CT: normative values for size and symmetry of the facial nerve canal, foramen ovale, pterygoid canal, and foramen rotundum. Surg Radiol Anat. 2013;35(1):19–24.

Singal A, Sahni D, Gupta T, Aggarwal A, Gupta AK. Anatomic variability of oval window as pertaining to stapes surgery. Surg Radiol Anat. 2020;42(3):329–35.

Todd NW, Creighton FX Jr. Malleus and incus: correlates of size. Ann Otol Rhinol Laryngol. 2013;122(1):60–5.

Ukkola-Pons E, Ayache D, Pons Y, Ratajczak M, Nioche C, Williams M. Oval window niche height: quantitative evaluation with CT before stapes surgery for otosclerosis. AJNR Am J Neuroradiol. 2013;34(5):1082–5.

Valvassori GE, Palacios E. Magnetic resonance imaging of the internal auditory canal. Top Magn Reson Imaging. 2000;11(1):52–65.

Valvassori GE, Garcia Morales F, Palacios E, Dobben GE. MR of the normal and abnormal internal auditory canal. AJNR Am J Neuroradiol. 1988;9(1):115–9.

Vijayasekaran S, Halsted MJ, Boston M, Meinzen-Derr J, Bardo DM, Greinwald J, Benton C. When is the vestibular aqueduct enlarged? A statistical analysis of the normative distribution of vestibular aqueduct size. AJNR Am J Neuroradiol. 2007;28(6):1133–8.

Yin D, Li C, Chen K, Hong J, Li J, Yang L, Zhang T, Dai P. Morphological characteristics of external auditory canal in congenital aural stenosis patients. Am J Otolaryngol. 2017;38(4):422–7.

Normative Measurements of the Skull Base on Imaging

4

Peleg M. Horowitz and
Daniel Thomas Ginat

4.1 Anterior Cranial Fossa

4.1.1 Ethmoid Roof

- Along with the fovea ethmoidalis, the cribriform plate forms the ethmoid roof.
- The cribriform plate is comprised of lateral (vertical) lamella and medial (horizontal) lamella on each side and contains multiple olfactory foramina that measure less than 1 mm in diameter, which are not readily discernible on computed tomography (CT).
- The depth of the olfactory fossa can be graded using the Keros classification (Fig. 4.1):
  - Type 1: has a depth of 1–3 mm
  - Type 2: has a depth of 4–7 mm (most common)
  - Type 3: has a depth of 8–16 mm (rare)

P. M. Horowitz
Department of Surgery, Section of Neurosurgery, University of Chicago, Chicago, IL, USA

D. T. Ginat (✉)
Department of Radiology, Section of Neuroradiology, University of Chicago, Chicago, IL, USA
e-mail: dtg1@uchicago.edu

© Springer Nature Switzerland AG 2021
D. T. Ginat (ed.), *Manual of Normative Measurements in Head and Neck Imaging*, https://doi.org/10.1007/978-3-030-50567-7_4

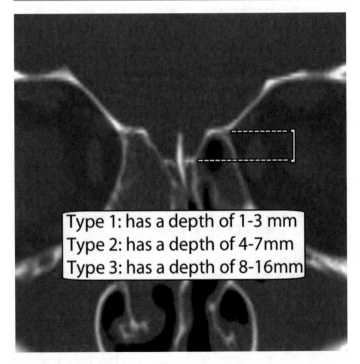

Type 1: has a depth of 1-3 mm
Type 2: has a depth of 4-7mm
Type 3: has a depth of 8-16mm

Fig. 4.1 Keros classification. Coronal computed tomography (CT) image shows depth of the olfactory fossa, measured from the fovea ethmoidalis to the medial lamella of the cribriform plate

Practical Implications

- The right half of the cribriform plate is usually lower than the left and the asymmetry can pose a potential risk for skull base injury and cerebrospinal fluid leak (Fig. 4.2).
- MRI should be obtained for further evaluation of possible cephalocele if dehiscence of the cribriform plate with opacification of the nasal cavity demonstrated are demonstrated on CT.

4.1.2 Crista Galli

- The crista galli is a bony structure that projects vertically into the intracranial cavity from the midline of the cribriform plate and is attached to the falx cerebri.

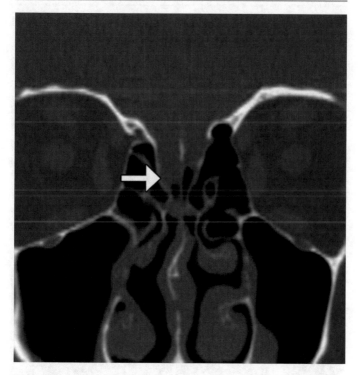

Fig. 4.2 Coronal computed tomography (CT) image shows an asymmetrically low right cribriform plate with dehiscence and what proved to be an encephalocele (arrow) in a patient with cerebrospinal fluid leak following endoscopic sinus surgery

- The typical dimensions of the crista galli include the following (Fig. 4.3):
    - 13 ± 2 mm in the anterior–posterior
    - 13 ± 3 mm in the cranial–caudal dimensions on average
    - 3 mm in thickness on the coronal plane (range: 1–8 mm)

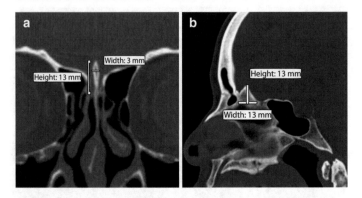

Fig. 4.3 Crista galli. Coronal (**a**) and sagittal (**b**) computed tomography (CT) images show the triangular bony structure along the superior aspect of the ethmoid roof with average dimensions denoted

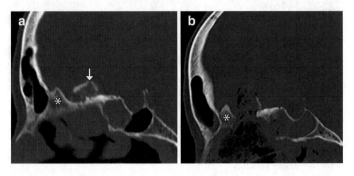

Fig. 4.4 Preoperative sagittal computed tomography (CT) image (**a**) shows a partially calcified olfactory groove meningioma (arrow) posterior to the crista galli (*). Postoperative sagittal CT image (**b**) shows interval resection of the mass via an endoscopic transcribriform approach with the anterior surgical margin marked by the posterior aspect of the crista galli (*)

Practical Implications

- Knowledge of the dimensions of the crista galli is relevant for planning resection of anterior cranial fossa tumors.
- Endoscopic transcribriform approach is the standard approach used, whereby the anterior limit of bone removal during this procedure is marked by boundary of the crista galli along with the posterior table of the frontal sinus (Fig. 4.4).

4.1.3   Olfactory Bulbs

- The olfactory bulbs are located in the olfactory grooves above the cribriform plates.
- Quantitative measurements of the olfactory bulb can be accurately performed via magnetic resonance imaging (MRI) using 2–3 mm interleaved coronal fast spin-echo T2-weighted scans with a long TR, a matrix size of 256 × 192, and a 12-cm field of view.
- The normal olfactory bulb diameter is 3 mm and the normal volume is 45 ± 12 mm^3 (Fig. 4.5).
- Abnormally small olfactory bulbs can be encountered with congenital anosmia, postinfectious or posttraumatic olfactory loss, and sinonasal-related olfactory dysfunction (Fig. 4.6).

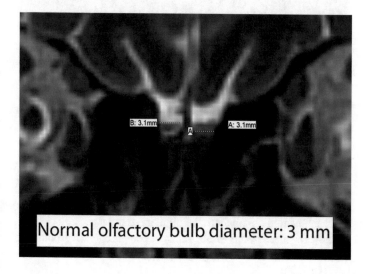

Fig. 4.5 Normal olfactory bulbs. Coronal T2-weighted magnetic resonance imaging (MRI) shows normal bilateral olfactory bulbs

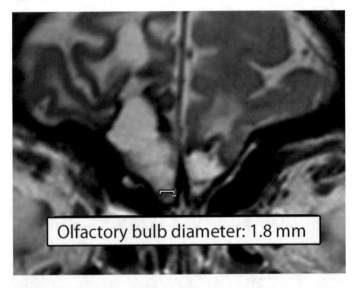

Olfactory bulb diameter: 1.8 mm

Fig. 4.6 Abnormal olfactory bulbs. Coronal T2-weighted magnetic resonance imaging (MRI) shows atrophic bilateral olfactory bulbs and frontal lobe encephalomalacia due to trauma

4.2 Middle Cranial Fossa and Pterygopalatine Fossa

4.2.1 Sella Turcica

- The sella turcica is a depression along the roof of the body of the sphenoid bone where the pituitary gland sits.
- Several measurements are relevant for preoperative planning for transsphenoidal surgery approaches to access the sella (Fig. 4.7):
  - Height ranges from 4 to 12 mm
  - Anteroposterior dimension ranges from 5 to 16 mm
  - Sellar face (line from the tuberculum sellae to the sellar–clival point): 13 mm

- Sellar prominence (longest perpendicular distance from the tuberculum–clival line to the most prominent point on the sellar floor convexity): 3 mm
- Planum sphenoidale length: 14 mm (range: 6–29 mm)
- Sellar angle: 112° (range: 71°–180°)
- Tuberculum sellae angle: 112° (range: 70°–154°)
- Sellar–clival angle: 117° (range: 65°–183°)

• The normal position of the chiasm is about 3–4 mm posterosuperior to the tuberculum.

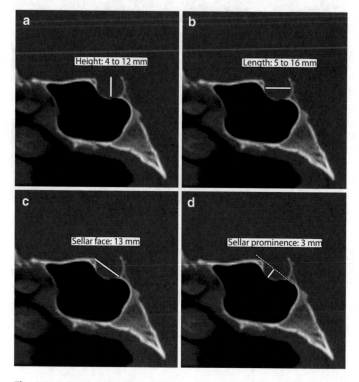

Fig. 4.7 Sella turcica. Sellar height (**a**), sellar anteroposterior dimension (**b**), sellar face (**c**), sellar prominence (**d**), length of planum sphenoidale (**e**), sellar angle (**f**), tuberculum sellae angle (**g**), sellar–clival angle (**h**)

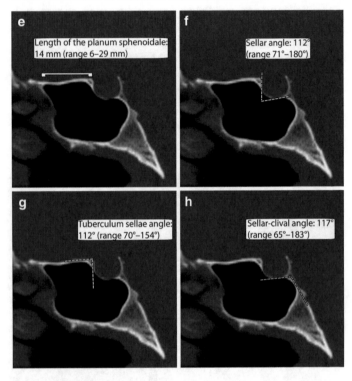

Fig. 4.7 (continued)

Practical Implications

- Compared with normal adults, patients with sellar lesions tend to have prominent sellar types, a more acute sellar angle, a more prominent sellar floor, and more acute tuberculum and sellar–clival angles.
- Larger sellar lesions, such as pituitary macroadenomas, also tend to cause expansion of the sella in one or more dimensions,

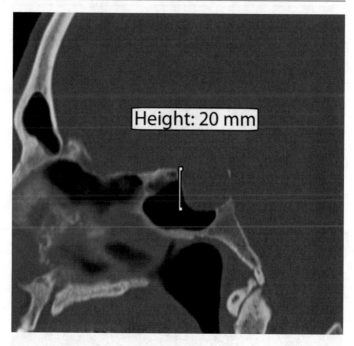

Fig. 4.8 Pituitary macroadenoma. Sagittal computed tomography (CT) image shows marked expansion of the sella caused by the pituitary tumor

and bony thinning of the sellar face, sometimes to the point of dehiscence (Fig. 4.8).
- A thick sellar face or incomplete pneumatization of the sphenoid sinus is more likely to require the use of a chisel or drill to expose the sella.

4.2.2   Pituitary Gland and Stalk

- The pituitary gland is situated in the sella of the sphenoid bone.
- The size varies substantially based on age and gender due to physiological neuroendocrine differences (Fig. 4.9):
    - The average height of the gland in children up to 12 years of age is 4 mm (range 2–6 mm).

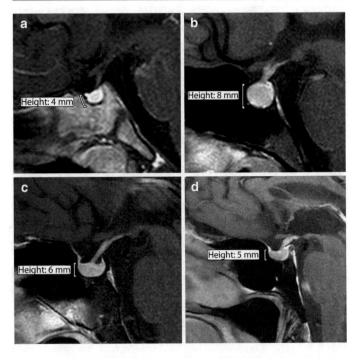

Fig. 4.9 Pituitary gland. Sagittal postcontrast MR images show the typical pituitary gland heights in an infant (**a**), adolescent female (**b**), middle aged adult (**c**), and elderly male (**d**)

- During adolescence, pituitary hypertrophy occurs in both sexes, but is more pronounced in girls, with a median height of the pituitary gland of 8–9 mm ± 1 mm and 6 ± 1 mm for girls and boys, respectively.
- The pituitary height peaks in the 20–29-age group and tends to decline with age. In females, the pituitary height can increase again in the 50–59-age group.
- The pituitary height in adult females (mean: 5.4 mm) is significantly greater than that in males (mean: 4.9 mm).

Practical Implications

- Besides the enhancement characteristics, the height of the pituitary gland is an important measurement for the detection of an intrasellar mass on MRI.
- Deviation of the pituitary stalk to either side should raise suspicion of a contralateral pituitary lesion.
- The superior margin of the gland can be convex in normal patients, but will usually not contact or displace the optic apparatus.
- Besides tumors, there can be diffuse enlargement of the pituitary gland, which can be caused by hyperplasia or hypophysitis (Fig. 4.10).

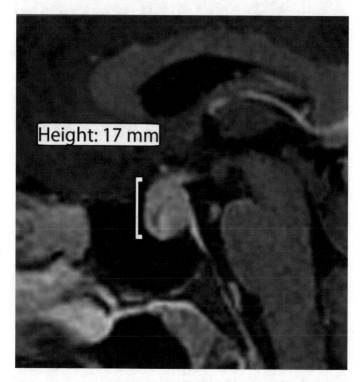

Fig. 4.10 Sagittal postcontrast T1-weighted magnetic resonance imaging (MRI) shows enlargement of the pituitary gland from hypophysitis caused by ipilimumab

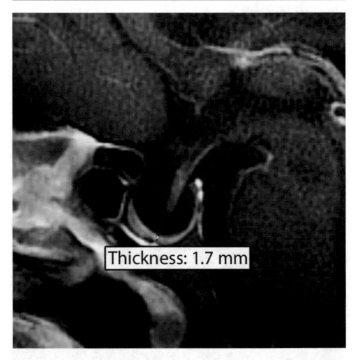

Thickness: 1.7 mm

Fig. 4.11 Partially empty sella. Sagittal postcontrast T1-weighted magnetic resonance imaging (MRI) shows an expanded sella with a thin pituitary gland that measures less than 2 mm in height

- A partially empty sella (more than 50% of the sella filled with cerebrospinal fluid and pituitary gland height measures up to 2 mm) can be found in cases of pituitary atrophy or pseudotumor cerebri (Fig. 4.11).

4.2.3 Meckel Cave

- The Meckel caves are cerebrospinal fluid-filled dural recesses located in the posteromedial portions of the middle cranial fossae, through which the trigeminal nerves pass.
- Contains the trigeminal nerve ganglion.

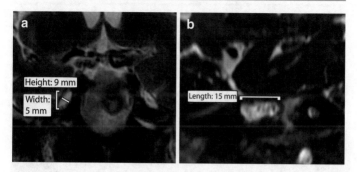

Fig. 4.12 Meckel cave. Coronal (**a**) and oblique sagittal (**b**) T2-weighted MR images show the typical dimensions of Meckel cave, where the rootlets of the trigeminal nerve are apparent

- Measures 4 × 9 mm wide at its opening and 15 mm in length (Fig. 4.12).
- The mean length of CN V proximal to the posterior margin of the Gasserian ganglion is 11.8 mm.
- The mean length of CN V1 is 19.4 mm; V2, 12.3 mm; and V3, 7.4 mm distal to the anterior margin of the ganglion.

Practical Implications
- Meckel caves can be narrowed in the setting of pseudotumor cerebri, measuring 2.5 mm in width on average (Fig. 4.13), or expanded in cases of trigeminal schwannomas and other tumors.

4.2.4 Carotid Sulcus

- The carotid sulcus is a groove in the body of the sphenoid bone and contains the cavernous segment of the internal carotid artery.
- The mean distance between the medial walls of the carotid sulcus is 16 ± 4 mm (Fig. 4.14).
- The mean paraclinoid intercarotid artery distance is 13 mm.

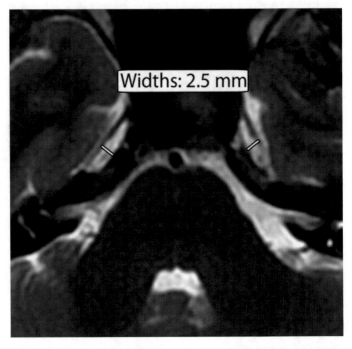

Fig. 4.13 Pseudotumor cerebri. Axial T2-weighted magnetic resonance imaging (MRI) in a patient shows narrowing of the bilateral Meckel caves

Practical Implications

- Being cognizant of the intercarotid distance is important to ensure a "safe-zone" for accessing the sella in all transsphenoidal approaches.
- Patients with pituitary macroadenomas tend to have a widened intercarotid distance.
- Preoperative assessment of the intercarotid distances is important for identifying constraints to endoscopic access of the skull base and avoiding inadvertent arterial injury (Fig. 4.15).

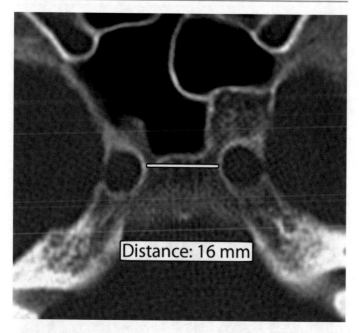

Fig. 4.14 Carotid sulcus. Axial computed tomography (CT) image depicts the average closest distance between the inner walls of the bilateral carotid sulci

4.2.5 Optic Canal

- Transmits the optic nerve and ophthalmic artery.
- Bounded medially by the body of the sphenoid bone, superiorly by the superior root of the lesser wing of the sphenoid bone, inferolaterally by the optic strut (i.e., the inferior root of the lesser wing of the sphenoid bone), and laterally by the anterior clinoid process.
- The optic canal is oriented at 45° with respect to the sagittal plane of the head.

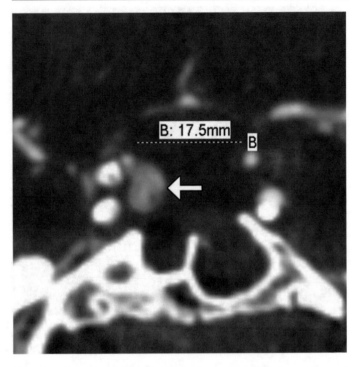

Fig. 4.15 Carotid pseudoaneurysm after transsphenoidal surgery. Coronal MIP CTA image shows an outpouching from the paraclinoid artery (arrow) and the paraclinoid intercarotid artery distance denoted

- The anterior end of the optic canal is narrower, with the intracranial and orbital openings measuring 4 × 6 mm and 5 × 6 mm on average, respectively (Fig. 4.16).
- The canal is 9 mm long on average (range: 8–12 mm).
- The optic canal volume decreases by nearly 5% per decade in adults.

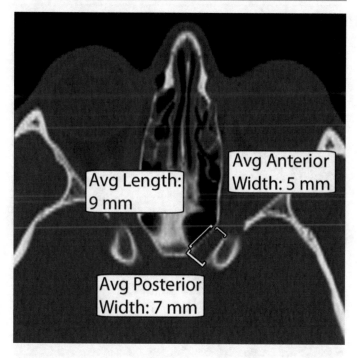

Fig. 4.16 Optic canal. Axial computed tomography (CT) image shows the average dimensions of the optic canal, which is wider posteriorly than anteriorly

Practical Implications
- Knowledge of the length of the optic canal is important for achieving adequate surgical decompression of the optic nerve.
- Dehiscence of the bone of the medial wall should also prompt caution during nasal approaches to the sella and tuberculum.
- Narrowing of the optic canals may require surgical decompression and can be caused by various conditions, such as Paget disease and osteopetrosis (Fig. 4.17).

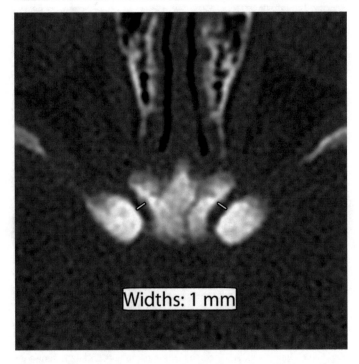

Fig. 4.17 Osteopetrosis. Axial computed tomography (CT) image in an infant shows marked narrowing of the bilateral optic nerve canals

4.2.6 Superior Orbital Fissure

- The superior orbital fissure is an oval canal in the anteromedial greater sphenoidal wing.
- Contents include the trochlear nerve, the frontal and lacrimal nerves (branches of V1), and the superior ophthalmic vein (listed lateral to medial), the oculomotor, nasociliary (branch of V1), and abducens nerves and roots from the ciliary ganglion, the inferior ophthalmic vein, orbital fat, and smooth muscle.
- The typical dimensions of the superior orbital fissure and associated landmarks include the following (Fig. 4.18):
  - The length ranges from 20 to 22 mm.

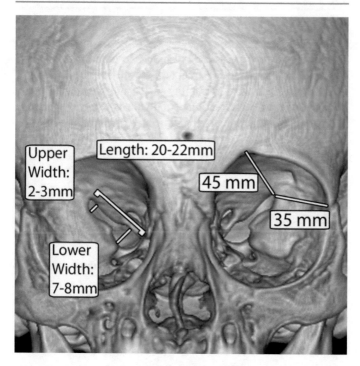

Fig. 4.18 Superior orbital fissure. 3D computed tomography (CT) image shows the oblong fissure, which is wider inferomedially than superolaterally, with average dimensions denoted on the right side. The average distances from the supraorbital notch/foramen and the frontozygomatic suture to the superior orbital fissure are denoted on the left side

- The superior and inferior widths are 2–3 mm and 7–8 mm, respectively.
- The average distance from the supraorbital notch/foramen to the superior orbital fissure is 45 mm.
- The average distance from the frontozygomatic suture to the superior orbital fissure is 35 mm.
- The trochlear nerve has an average diameter of 0.5 mm.

Practical Implications

- It is desirable to preserve the thin portions of the greater wing inferior to the superior orbital fissure in order to avoid exposure of the dura during lateral orbital wall decompression.
- There is substantial variability in the morphometrics of the superior orbital fissures among individuals, which underscores the need for individualized preoperative imaging assessment.

4.2.7 Foramen Rotundum

- Foramen rotundum extends from the middle cranial fossa to the pterygopalatine fossa.
- The foramen transmits the maxillary division of the trigeminal nerve.
- The typical dimensions of the foramen rotundum and associated landmarks are as follows (Fig. 4.19):
  - Mean diameter: 3 mm (standard deviation: 0.4 mm)
  - Foramen rotundum to midline axis: 19 mm (standard deviation: 2 mm)
  - Rotundum angle: 147°

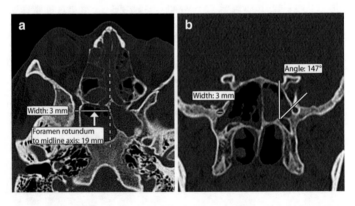

Fig. 4.19 Foramen rotundum. Axial (**a**) and coronal (**b**) computed tomography (CT) images depict the typical dimensions of foramen rotundum and the rotundum angle

Practical Implications
- The distances of the foramen rotundum to the Vidian canal are symmetrical in different axes, which can help localize the foramen rotundum in relation to Vidian canal and facilitate its safe identification during endoscopic surgery.

4.2.8   Foramen Ovale

- Foramen ovale connects the middle cranial fossa with the infratemporal fossa, transmits the mandibular division of the trigeminal nerve.
- The foramen can have various shapes including oval, almond, round, and slit. The predominant shape is oval, with an average aspect ratio of 2.1 and roundness of 0.5.
- Several measurements to consider include the following (Fig. 4.20):
  - Average cross-sectional dimension: 4 × 7 mm (range: 2 × 5 to 8 × 7 mm)
  - The angle formed between the long axis of the foramen ovale and the coronal plane averages 35° ± 10° (mean ± SD)
  - The average distance from foramen ovale to the second molar is 52 mm in males and 49 mm in females

Practical Implications
- Foramen ovale allows access to the trigeminal nerve and knowledge of its position and measurements are relevant for stereotactic neurosurgical planning and successful cannulation.
- As with other skull base foramina, enlargement of the foramen ovale can be a sign of tumor, such as in the form of perineural spread, which may be otherwise inconspicuous on CT and may prompt further work up with MRI (Fig. 4.21).

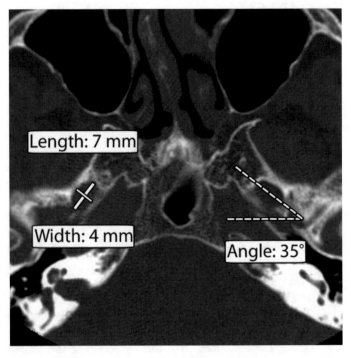

Fig. 4.20 Foramen ovale. Axial computed tomography (CT) image depicts the average dimensions and orientation of foramen ovale

4.2.9   Foramen Spinosum

- Foramen spinosum is an opening in the greater wing of the sphenoid bone and lies posterolateral to foramen ovale.
- Contains the middle meningeal artery, the middle meningeal vein(s), and a recurrent branch of the mandibular nerve (nervus spinosus).
- The average width: 2 mm (range: 1.5–3.0 mm) and the typical length: 2–4 mm (Fig. 4.22).

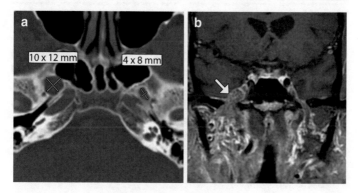

Fig. 4.21 Perineural tumor spread. Axial computed tomography (CT) image (**a**) shows asymmetric enlargement of the right foramen ovale. The corresponding coronal postcontrast magnetic resonance imaging (MRI) (**b**) shows perineural tumor (arrow) extending through the right foramen ovale in a patient with adenoid cystic carcinoma

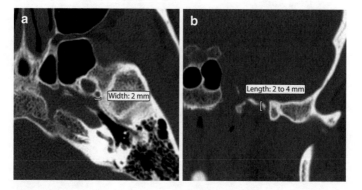

Fig. 4.22 Foramen spinosum. Axial (**a**) and coronal (**b**) computed tomography (CT) images depict the typical dimensions of foramen spinosum

Practical Implications

- Foramen spinosum is a landmark for middle cranial fossa microsurgery, particularly for hemostasis, but is sometimes absent or continuous with foramen ovale.

4.2.10 Vidian (Pterygoid) Canal

- The Vidian canal is situated between the pterygoid process and the sphenoid sinus. It is directed forward and medially and connects the foramen lacerum with the pterygopalatine fossa.
- Transmits the Vidian artery that arises from the internal maxillary artery and the Vidian nerve that carries parasympathetic fibers to the sphenopalatine ganglion in the pterygopalatine fossa.
- The width of the canal varies along its length, widening as it extends forward.
- The typical dimensions of the Vidian canal and are as follows (Fig. 4.23):
  - The average width of its anterior opening is 2.5 mm, versus 1 mm for the posterior opening.
  - The mean length of the Vidian canal is 14–18 mm (range: 10–23 mm).

Practical Implications
- The Vidian canal is an important landmark in endoscopic transpterygoid approaches, and reliably leads to the carotid canal.
- The amount of bone that needs to be drilled during the approach will be related to the length and degree of pneumatization.
- Drilling clockwise inferior to superior around the Vidian canal allows for safe petrous internal carotid artery localization in most cases.

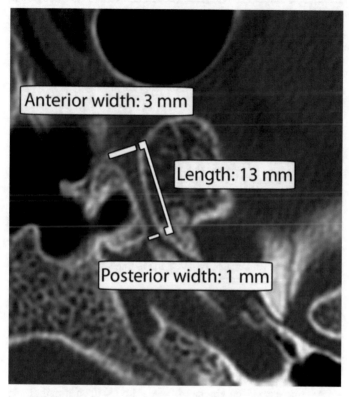

Fig. 4.23 Vidian canal. Axial computed tomography (CT) image depicts the typical length of the Vidian canal, which is wider anteriorly than posteriorly

4.2.11 Foramen Vesalius

- Foramen Vesalius is an inconsistent channel located in the greater sphenoid wing posterior to the foramen rotundum.
- The foramen transmits a small vein that connects the cavernous sinus with the pterygoid venous plexus.

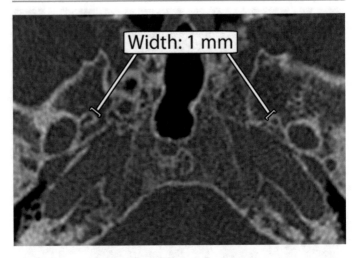

Fig. 4.24 Foramen Vesalius. Axial CT image shows the typical size of the foramen, which is symmetric

- The foramen average width is 1.0 mm (standard deviation: 0.1 mm) and the average length is 1.7 mm (standard deviation: 0.7 mm) (Fig. 4.24).

Practical Implications
- Asymmetry of the channel is often the result of a pathologic process rather than a normal variant.

4.2.12 Pterygopalatine Fossa

- The pterygopalatine fossa is an inverted pyramid-shaped space bounded by the junction of the maxilla, palatine, and sphenoid bones.
- Contains fat, the pterygopalatine ganglion, the maxillary division (V2) of the trigeminal nerve and its branches (zygomatic nerve, posterior superior alveolar nerve, and the infraorbital nerve), the Vidian nerve, the distal branches of the maxillary artery, and emissary veins.

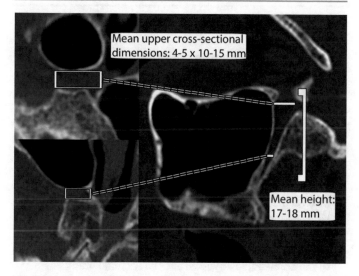

Fig. 4.25 Pterygopalatine fossa. The pterygopalatine fossa is larger superiorly than inferiorly as shown on the axial (left) and sagittal (right) computed tomography (CT) images

- In cross-section, the pterygopalatine fossa appears as a small oval or rectangular space with typical dimensions of 4–5 × 10–15 mm in the upper region and an average height of the pterygopalatine fossa is 17–18 mm (range 10–25 mm) (Fig. 4.25).
- The pterygopalatine fossa communicates with the infratemporal fossa via the pterygomaxillary fissure and communicates with the nasal cavity via the sphenopalatine foramen, which measures an average of 5 mm in the vertical dimension (range: 3–7 mm).

Practical Implications
- The anatomy of the pterygopalatine fossa is pertinent to maxillary nerve block procedures at the foramen rotundum.
- A narrow pterygomaxillary fissure can be an obstacle for such procedures, while an enlarged pterygopalatine fossa may indicate the presence of tumor, such as from perineural spread.

4.3   Posterior Fossa

4.3.1   Jugular Foramen and Bulb

- The jugular foramen is located between the occipital bone and the petrous part of the temporal bone.
- The foramen consists of a smaller anteromedial portion (pars nervosa) and a larger posterolateral portion (pars vascularis), which are separated by a complete or incomplete fibrous or bony septum.
- The pars nervosa contains the glossopharyngeal nerve and the inferior petrosal sinus as it courses between the cavernous sinus and jugular bulb.
- The pars vascularis contains the internal jugular vein, the vagus nerve, the spinal accessory nerve, and the meningeal branches of the ascending pharyngeal and the occipital artery.
- The jugular foramen varies greatly in size, but averages 1.5 cm in length and 1.0 cm in width (Fig. 4.26).
- The pars nervosa averages about 5 mm in width.
- In two-third of individuals, the right jugular foramen is larger than the left jugular foramen.
- Average cross-sectional dimensions are 7–8 × 23–24 mm.
- The diameters of CN IX, X, and XI are 2.3, 4.6, and 3.5 mm, respectively.
- The mean distance between the mastoid tip and jugular foramen is 21 mm (range: 11–28 mm).
- The average jugular bulb height (distance from jugular dome to intersection with sigmoid sinus): 8 mm (range: 4–12 mm) (Fig. 4.27).

Practical Implications
- Asymmetry of the jugular foramen usually relates to normal underlying asymmetry of the venous drainage system through the transverse and sigmoid sinuses.
- Enlargement of the jugular foramen with erosion can be associated with tumors, such as paragangliomas (Fig. 4.28).

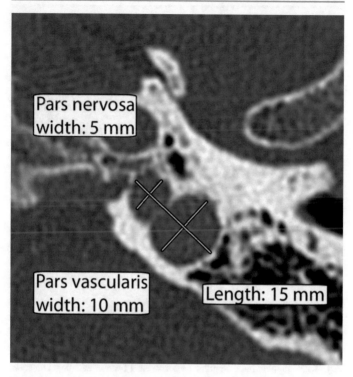

Fig. 4.26 Jugular foramen. Axial computed tomography (CT) image depicts the typical dimensions of the endocranial aspect of the jugular foramen

- Enlargement of the jugular foramen without erosion is probably of pathologic significance if the sum of its length, the width of the pars vascularis, and the width of the pars nervosa is 20 mm greater than that of the opposite side.
- A high-riding jugular bulb can be defined as a jugular bulb that is at or above the level of the basal turn of the cochlea, within 2 mm of the internal auditory canal, or up to the level of the superior tympanic annulus.

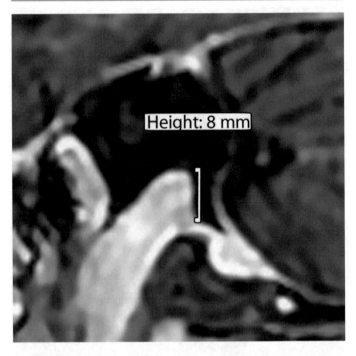

Fig. 4.27 Jugular bulb. Sagittal postcontrast T1-weighted magnetic resonance imaging (MRI) shows the height of the jugular bulb from its dome to the junction with the sigmoid sinus

4.3.2 Hypoglossal Canal

- The hypoglossal canal is located on the anterior aspect of the occipital bone, inferolateral to the inferior edge of the clivus and 8 mm inferomedial to the jugular foramen.
- Contains the hypoglossal venous plexus and in 45% of cases the meningeal branch of the ascending pharyngeal artery.
- The jugular tubercle is a bony protuberance from the inferolateral margin of the clivus that projects posterosuperiorly over the hypoglossal canal.

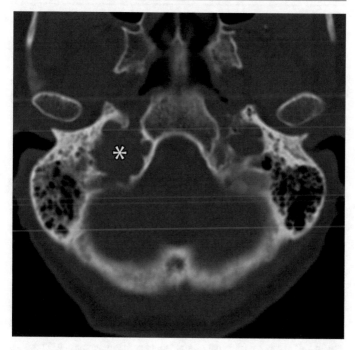

Fig. 4.28 Jugular foramen paraganglioma. Axial computed tomography (CT) image shows asymmetric widening of the right jugular foramen (*) with erosions of the margins

- The intracranial opening of the foramen measures 6 × 4 mm cross-section on average, whereas the extracranial opening is narrower, at 5 × 3 mm, but can vary by up to 2 mm in each dimension, and the canal length is typically 7–9 mm (Fig. 4.29).
- The typical diameter of the hypoglossal nerve is 1.6–1.7 mm.
- The mean length of the jugular tubercle is 14 mm (range: 10–28 mm) (Fig. 4.30).
- The average distance between the jugular foramen and hypoglossal canal is 2.5 mm (range: 2–4 mm).

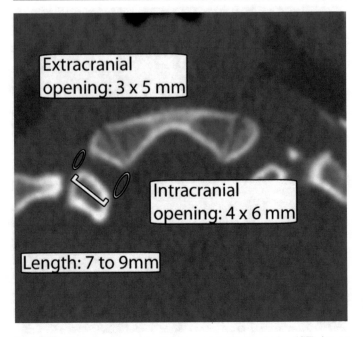

Fig. 4.29 Hypoglossal canal. Axial computed tomography (CT) image shows the typical dimensions of the canal

Practical Implications
- The hypoglossal canal is often considered to be the medial limit in transcondylar exposures of the posterolateral skull base with "far lateral" approaches.
- Such approaches allow for access to pathology at the vertebrobasilar junction, such as aneurysms and anterolateral foramen magnum for tumors of the lower clivus.
- Resection of the occipital condyle beyond the hypoglossal canal may cause occipitocervical instability requiring fusion.

4.3.3 Clivus

- The clivus comprises the central part of the base of the skull and has a wedge-shaped configuration on sagittal sections.

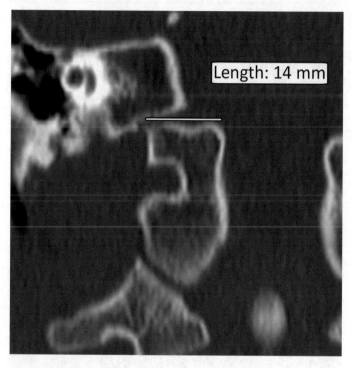

Fig. 4.30 Jugular tubercle. Coronal computed tomography (CT) image denotes the average length of the jugular tubercle

- In adults, the mean normal clival dimensions include the following (Fig. 4.31):
  - Intracranial clivus length from the top of the dorsum sellae to the basion: 43–45 mm (range: 37–54 mm)
  - Extracranial clival length: 28 ± 3 mm
  - Narrowest clival width: 20 ± 2 mm
  - Clival widest diameter (the widest diameter between the anterolateral left and right occipital condyles): 33 ± 3 mm
- The longitudinal diameter of extracranial clivus is 25.9 ± 2.6 mm. The narrowest diameter of the clivus is 12.8 ± 1.1 mm, the distance between the left and right hypoglossal canal is 32.7 ± 2.1 mm at its widest part.

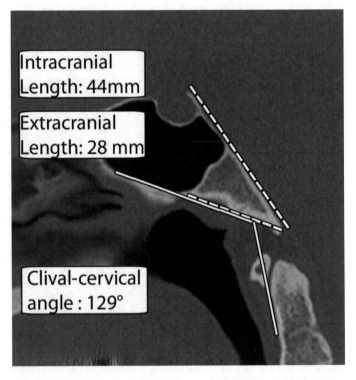

Fig. 4.31 Clivus. Sagittal computed tomography (CT) images shows the average dimensions of the clivus in an adult

- In children, the mean normal clival dimensions include:
  - Clival length: 29 mm
  - Widest diameter: 29 mm
  - Narrowest diameter: 17 mm
  - Fissure distance: 21 mm
  - Putative screw length: 10 mm
  - Clival–cervical angle (the angle between the tangent of the extracranial clivus and the tangent of the anterior cervical vertebrae in the midsagittal plane):129° ± 6°

Practical Implications

- Screws can be inserted into the clivus for craniovertebral fixation and imaging is important for determining screw length and angle of screw placement.
- Clival hypoplasia can be a component of congenital conditions, such as CHARGE syndrome and Chiari type 1 malformation.

4.3.4 Posterior Fossa

- The mean height of posterior fossa measured as the perpendicular distance between Twining's line (from internal occipital protuberance to posterior clinoid) and McRae line (from basion to opisthion) is 3.5 ± 0.4 cm based on CT (Fig. 4.32).

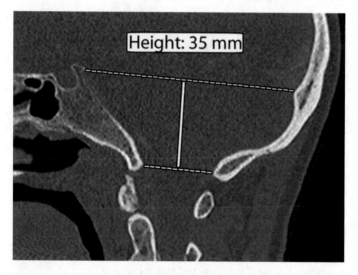

Fig. 4.32 Posterior fossa height. The height of the posterior fossa is measured between the Twining's line and McRae's line

- The anteroposterior diameter of the posterior fossa can be measured along a line parallel to the plane of the foramen magnum, from the top of the dorsum sella and is normally 75 mm on average.
- The mean volume of posterior fossa is 158 ± 28 cm^3.

Practical Implications
- Many conditions are associated with abnormal size of the posterior fossa, including Arnold–Chiari malformation, myelomeningocele, Dandy–Walker malformation, and platybasia.
- Neuroimaging is useful for assessing associated anomalies, such as with the cerebellum, in congenital cases with a small or large posterior fossa (Fig. 4.33).

4.3.5 Cerebellar Tonsil Position

- The range of cerebellar tonsil position has a nearly normal distribution in the population.
- The average height of the tonsil decreases slightly with age until young adulthood and increases thereafter.
- Generally, extension of the tonsils below the foramen magnum is considered normal up to 3 mm, borderline between 3 and 5 mm, and abnormal beyond 5 mm (Fig. 4.34).

Practical Implications
- Chiari type 1 malformation can be diagnosed on imaging based on the extent of tonsil location below the foramen magnum by at least 5 or 6 mm (Fig. 4.35), along with abnormal morphology of the tonsil, which tends to be pointed, and in some cases there is an accompanying syrinx.
- Inferior cerebellar tonsil herniation can also be encountered in cases of cerebellar edema and tumors (Fig. 4.36).

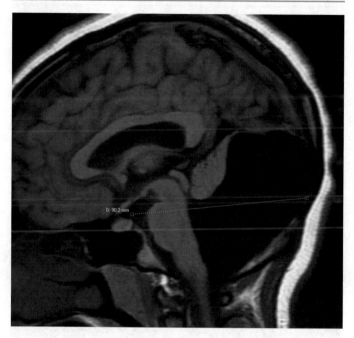

Fig. 4.33 Dandy–Walker malformation. Sagittal T1-weighted magnetic resonance imaging (MRI) shows an enlarged posterior fossa with a dysplastic cerebellum

4.3.6   Foramen Magnum

- The foramen magnum is an opening in the occipital bone with borders formed anteriorly by the inferior aspect of the downward-sloping clivus, laterally on both sides by the jugular tubercles, and posteriorly by the edge of the squamous part of the occipital bone.
- Contents include the medulla oblongata, meninges, spinal root of cranial nerve XI, vertebral arteries, anterior and posterior spinal arteries, the tectorial membrane, and alar ligaments.
- Can have a variety of shapes: round, oval, egg-shaped, tetragonal, pentagonal, hexagonal, and irregular.

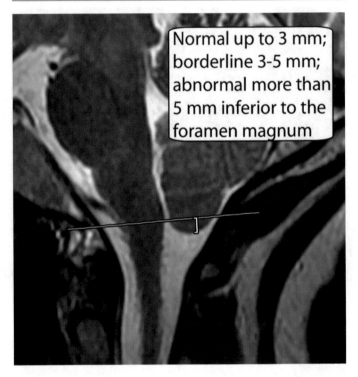

Fig. 4.34 Sagittal T2-weighted magnetic resonance imaging (MRI) denotes the range of cerebellar tonsil positions with respect to the basion–opisthion line

- The dimensions of the foramen magnum in adults include the following (Fig. 4.37):
  - The anteroposterior diameter is 35–40 mm in males, with a mean of 37 mm, and 30–35 mm, in females with a mean of 33 mm
  - The transverse diameter is 26–34 mm in males, with a mean of 30 mm, and between 26 and 31.75 mm in females, with a mean of 30 mm
  - The mean area of foramen magnum in males is 877 mm^2 in males and 777 mm^2 in females

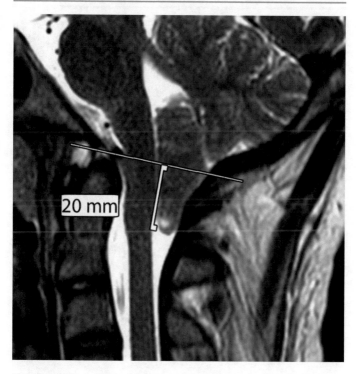

Fig. 4.35 Chiari malformation. Sagittal T2-weighted magnetic resonance imaging (MRI) shows extension of a cerebellar tonsil 20 mm inferior to the foramen magnum with pointed morphology

Practical Implications

- Achondroplasia is associated with foramen magnum stenosis, often in conjunction with basilar invagination (Fig. 4.38).
- Stenosis of foramen magnum can cause brainstem compression manifested by respiratory complications, lower cranial nerve dysfunctions, upper and lower extremity paresis, hypo- or hypertonia, hyperreflexia, or clonus.

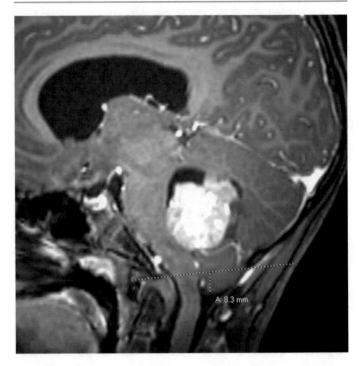

A: 8.3 mm

Fig. 4.36 Cerebellar tonsil herniation. Sagittal postcontrast T1-weighted magnetic resonance imaging (MRI) shows inferior cerebellar tonsil extension through the foramen magnum in a child with an ependymoma

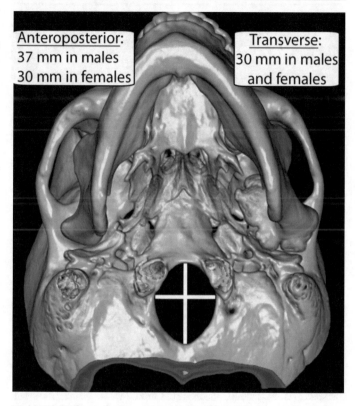

Fig. 4.37 Foramen magnum. Average lengths and widths in normal adult male and females

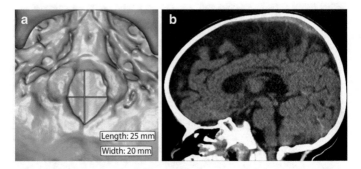

Fig. 4.38 Achondroplasia. 3D computed tomography (CT) rendering (**a**) shows the dimensions of a stenotic foramen magnum. Sagittal CT image (**b**) shows that mild basilar invagination further narrows the foramen magnum. Also note the characteristic frontal bossing

Further Reading

Aboulezz AO, Sartor K, Geyer CA, Gado MH. Position of cerebellar tonsils in the normal population and in patients with Chiari malformation: a quantitative approach with MR imaging. J Comput Assist Tomogr. 1985;9(6):1033–6.

Aydin S, Hanimoglu H, Tanriverdi T, Yentur E, Kaynar MY. Chiari type I malformations in adults: a morphometric analysis of the posterior cranial fossa. Surg Neurol. 2005;64(3):237–41.

Barkovich AJ, Wippold FJ, Sherman JL, Citrin CM. Significance of cerebellar tonsillar position on MR. AJNR Am J Neuroradiol. 1986;7(5):795–9.

Beden U, Edizer M, Elmali M, Icten N, Gungor I, Sullu Y, Erkan D. Surgical anatomy of the deep lateral orbital wall. Eur J Ophthalmol. 2007;17(3):281–6.

Berlis A, Putz R, Schumacher M. Direct and CT measurements of canals and foramina of the skull base. Br J Radiol. 1992;65(776):653–61.

Caldemeyer KS, Mathews VP, Azzarelli B, Smith RR. The jugular foramen: a review of anatomy, masses, and imaging characteristics. Radiographics. 1997;17(5):1123–39.

Chen J, Xiao J. Morphological study of the pterygoid canal with high-resolution CT. Int J Clin Exp Med. 2015;8(6):9484–90. eCollection 2015.

Coelho DH, Pence TS, Abdel-Hamid M, Costanzo RM. Cribriform plate width is highly variable within and between subjects. Auris Nasus Larynx. 2018;45(5):1000–5.

Degnan AJ, Levy LM. Narrowing of Meckel's cave and cavernous sinus and enlargement of the optic nerve sheath in Pseudotumor Cerebri. J Comput Assist Tomogr. 2011;35(2):308–12.

Doyle AJ. Optic chiasm position on MR images. AJNR Am J Neuroradiol. 1990;11(3):553–5.

Ebner FH, Kuerschner V, Dietz K, Bueltmann E, Naegele T, Honegger J. Reduced intercarotid artery distance in acromegaly: pathophysiologic considerations and implications for transsphenoidal surgery. Surg Neurol. 2009;72(5):456–60; discussion 4.

Edwards B, Wang JM, Iwanaga J, Loukas M, Tubbs RS. Cranial nerve foramina part I: a review of the anatomy and pathology of cranial nerve foramina of the anterior and middle fossa. Cureus. 2018;10(2):e2172. https://doi.org/10.7759/cureus.2172.

Edwards B, Wang JM, Iwanaga J, Loukas M, Tubbs RS. Cranial nerve foramina: part II—a review of the anatomy and pathology of cranial nerve foramina of the posterior cranial fossa. Cureus. 2018c;10(4):e2500.

Elster AD, Chen MY, Williams DW 3rd, Key LL. Pituitary gland: MR imaging of physiologic hypertrophy in adolescence. Radiology. 1990;174(3 Pt 1):681–5.

Ginat DT, Ellika SK, Corrigan J. Multi-detector-row computed tomography imaging of variant skull base foramina. J Comput Assist Tomogr. 2013;37(4):481–5.

Ginsberg LE, Pruett SW, Chen MY, Elster AD. Skull-base foramina of the middle cranial fossa: reassessment of normal variation with high-resolution CT. AJNR Am J Neuroradiol. 1994;15(2):283–91.

Inal M, Muluk NB, Arikan OK, Şahin S. Is there a relationship between optic canal, foramen rotundum, and vidian canal? J Craniofac Surg. 2015;26(4):1382–8.

Janjua RM, Al-Mefty O, Densler DW, Shields CB. Dural relationships of Meckel cave and lateral wall of the cavernous sinus. Neurosurg Focus. 2008;25(6):E2.

Jiang PF, Dai XY, Lv Y, Liu S, Mu XY. Imaging study on the optic canal using sixty four-slice spiral computed tomography. Int J Clin Exp Med. 2015;8(11):21247–51.

Kalthur SG, Padmashali S, Gupta C, Dsouza AS. Anatomic study of the occipital condyle and its surgical implications in transcondylar approach. J Craniovertebr Junction Spine. 2014;5(2):71–7.

Kanodia G, Parihar V, Yadav YR, Bhatele PR, Sharma D. Morphometric analysis of posterior fossa and foramen magnum. J Neurosci Rural Pract. 2012;3(3):261–6. https://doi.org/10.4103/0976-3147.102602.

Keles B, Semaan MT, Fayad JN. The medial wall of the jugular foramen: a temporal bone anatomic study. Otolaryngol Head Neck Surg. 2009;141(3):401–7.

Keros P. On the practical value of differences in the level of the lamina cribrosa of the ethmoid [in German]. Z Laryngol Rhinol Otol. 1962;41:808–13.

Kim HS, Kim DI, Chung IH. High-resolution CT of the pterygopalatine fossa and its communications. Neuroradiology. 1996;38(Suppl 1):S120–6.

Koenigsberg RA, Vakil N, Hong TA, Htaik T, Faerber E, Maiorano T, Dua M, Faro S, Gonzales C. Evaluation of platybasia with MR imaging. AJNR Am J Neuroradiol. 2005;26(1):89–92.

Lee JM, Ransom E, Lee JY, Palmer JN, Chiu AG. Endoscopic anterior skull base surgery: intraoperative considerations of the crista galli. Skull Base. 2011;21(2):83–6.

Lega BC, Kramer DR, Newman JG, Lee JY. Morphometric measurements of the anterior skull base for endoscopic transoral and transnasal approaches. Skull Base. 2011;21(1):65–70.

Lyrtzis C, Piagkou M, Gkioka A, Anastasopoulos N, Apostolidis S, Natsis K. Foramen magnum, occipital condyles and hypoglossal canals morphometry: anatomical study with clinical implications. Folia Morphol (Warsz). 2017;76(3):446–57.

Manjila S, Bazil T, Kay M, Udayasankar UK, Semaan M. Jugular bulb and skull base pathologies: proposal for a novel classification system for jugular bulb positions and microsurgical implications. Neurosurg Focus. 2018;45(1):E5.

Mascarella MA, Forghani R, Di Maio S, Sirhan D, Zeitouni A, Mohr G, Tewfik MA. Indicators of a reduced intercarotid artery distance in patients undergoing endoscopic transsphenoidal surgery. J Neurol Surg B Skull Base. 2015;76(3):195–201.

Mason EC, Hudgins PA, Pradilla G, Oyesiku NM, Solares CA. Radiographic analysis of the vidian canal and its utility in petrous internal carotid artery localization. Oper Neurosurg (Hagerstown). 2018;15(5):577–83.

Mintelis A, Sameshima T, Bulsara KR, Gray L, Friedman AH, Fukushima T. Jugular tubercle: morphometric analysis and surgical significance. J Neurosurg. 2006;105(5):753–7.

Mohebbi A, Rajaeih S, Safdarian M, Omidian P. The sphenoid sinus, foramen rotundum and vidian canal: a radiological study of anatomical relationships. Braz J Otorhinolaryngol. 2017;83(4):381–7.

Pandolfo I, Gaeta M, Blandino A, Longo M. The radiology of the pterygoid canal: normal and pathologic findings. AJNR Am J Neuroradiol. 1987;8(3):479–83.

Pang J, Hou S, Liu M, et al. Puncture of foramen ovale cranium in computed tomography three-dimensional reconstruction. J Craniofac Surg. 2012;23:1457–9.

Rombaux P, Grandin C, Duprez T. How to measure olfactory bulb volume and olfactory sulcus depth? B-ENT. 2009;5(Suppl 13):53–60.

Sathyanarayana HP, Kailasam V, Chitharanjan AB. Sella turcica—its importance in orthodontics and craniofacial morphology. Dent Res J (Isfahan). 2013;10(5):571–5.

Satogami N, Miki Y, Koyama T, Kataoka M, Togashi K. Normal pituitary stalk: high-resolution MR imaging at 3T. AJNR Am J Neuroradiol. 2010;31(2):355–9.

Sepahdari AR, Mong S. Skull base CT: normative values for size and symmetry of the facial nerve canal, foramen ovale, pterygoid canal, and foramen rotundum. Surg Radiol Anat. 2013;35(1):19–24.

Smith BW, Strahle J, Bapuraj JR, Muraszko KM, Garton HJ, Maher CO. Distribution of cerebellar tonsil position: implications for understanding Chiari malformation. J Neurosurg. 2013;119(3):812–9.

Smoker WR, Khanna G. Imaging the craniocervical junction. Childs Nerv Syst. 2008;24(10):1123–45.

Solares CA, Lee WT, Batra PS, Citardi MJ. Lateral lamella of the cribriform plate: software-enabled computed tomographic analysis and its clinical relevance in skull base surgery. Arch Otolaryngol Head Neck Surg. 2008;134(3):285–9. https://doi.org/10.1001/archotol.134.3.285.

Stojcev Stajcić L, Gacić B, Popović N, Stajcić Z. Anatomical study of the pterygopalatine fossa pertinent to the maxillary nerve block at the foramen rotundum. Int J Oral Maxillofac Surg. 2010;39(5):493–6.

Suzuki M, Takashima T, Kadoya M, Konishi H, Kameyama T, Yoshikawa J, Gabata T, Arai K, Tamura S, Yamamoto T, et al. Height of normal pituitary gland on MR imaging: age and sex differentiation. J Comput Assist Tomogr. 1990;14(1):36–9.

Tashi S, Purohit BS, Becker M, Mundada P. The pterygopalatine fossa: imaging anatomy, communications, and pathology revisited. Insights Imaging. 2016;7(4):589–99.

Terano T, Seya A, Tamura Y, Yoshida S, Hirayama T. Characteristics of the pituitary gland in elderly subjects from magnetic resonance images: relationship to pituitary hormone secretion. Clin Endocrinol. 1996;45(3):273–9.

Tsunoda A, Okuda O, Sato K. MR height of the pituitary gland as a function of age and sex: especially physiological hypertrophy in adolescence and in climacterium. AJNR Am J Neuroradiol. 1997;18(3):551–4.

Verma R, Kumar S, Rai AM, Mansoor I, Mehra RD. The anatomical perspective of human occipital condyle in relation to the hypoglossal canal, condylar canal, and jugular foramen and its surgical significance. J Craniovertebr Junction Spine. 2016;7(4):243–9.

Vescan AD, Snyderman CH, Carrau RL, Mintz A, Gardner P, Branstetter B 4th, Kassam AB. Vidian canal: analysis and relationship to the internal carotid artery. Laryngoscope. 2007;117(8):1338–42.

Zacharek MA, Han JK, Allen R, Weissman JL, Hwang PH. Sagittal and coronal dimensions of the ethmoid roof: a radioanatomic study. Am J Rhinol. 2005;19(4):348–52.

Zada G, Agarwalla PK, Mukundan S Jr, Dunn I, Golby AJ, Laws ER Jr. The neurosurgical anatomy of the sphenoid sinus and sellar floor in endoscopic transsphenoidal surgery. J Neurosurg. 2011;114(5):1319–30.

Normative Measurements of the Craniocervical Junction on Imaging

5

Daniel Thomas Ginat and
Peleg M. Horowitz

5.1 Craniocervical Lines, Angles, and Measurements

- Chamberlain line (Fig. 5.1): Extends from the posterior margin of hard palate to opisthion (Fig. 5.1). The tip of the odontoid should be no more than 5 mm above this line and the anterior arch of C1 typically lies below this. Clivus height is the distance of the basion above Chamberlain line. These radiographic indicators are used to detect basilar invagination or impression. The McGregor line is an alternative to the Chamberlain line for the evaluation of basilar invagination when the opisthion is not apparent on radiographs and extends from the posterior margin of hard palate to inferior aspect of the occipital bone.

D. T. Ginat (✉)
Department of Radiology, Section of Neuroradiology,
University of Chicago, Chicago, IL, USA
e-mail: dtg1@uchicago.edu

P. M. Horowitz
Department of Surgery, Section of Neurosurgery, University of Chicago,
Chicago, IL, USA

© Springer Nature Switzerland AG 2021
D. T. Ginat (ed.), *Manual of Normative Measurements in Head and Neck Imaging*, https://doi.org/10.1007/978-3-030-50567-7_5

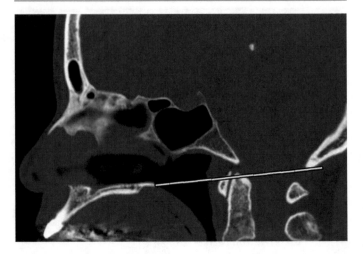

Fig. 5.1 Sagittal computed tomography (CT) image shows the Chamberlain line

- Wackenheim clivus baseline (Fig. 5.2): Line extrapolated inferiorly along dorsal surface of the clivus. The line should fall tangent to or intersect the posterior third of the odontoid and is used to detect basilar invagination or impression.

- McRae line (Fig. 5.3): Line from the basion to opisthion. The normal position of the tip of dens is 5 mm below this line and is used to detect basilar invagination or impression.

- Palatal line (Fig. 5.4): Line drawn parallel to the superior edge of the palatine process starting posterior to the anterior nasal spine. The normal mean height of the odontoid over the palatine line is 3.5 mm (range: 0–19.0 mm). In cases with platybasia, the mean is 15.5 mm (range: 7–26.0 mm).

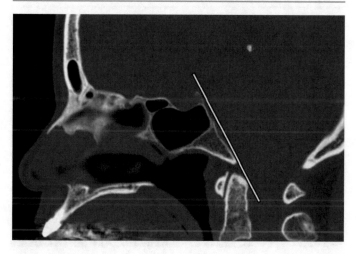

Fig. 5.2 Sagittal computed tomography (CT) image shows the Wackenheim clivus baseline

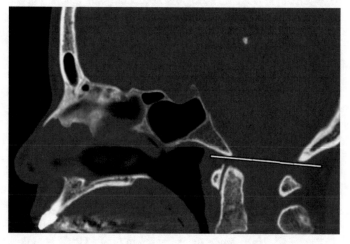

Fig. 5.3 Sagittal computed tomography (CT) image shows the McRae line

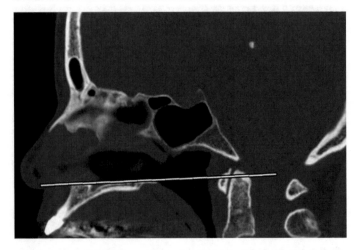

Fig. 5.4 Sagittal computed tomography (CT) image shows the palatal line

- Basal angle (Fig. 5.5): Angle subtended by the junction of the nasion–tuberculum and tuberculum–basion tangents. The normal ranges are as follows:
  - 116°–118°, 95% confidence limits for adults
  - 113°–115°, 95% confidence limits for children
  - Platybasia >143°
  A modified version of the basal angle formed by a line from the nasion and the center of the pituitary fossa and a line joining the anterior border of the foramen magnum result in the following normal mean angles:
  - 129° ± 6° for adults
  - 127° ± 5° for children

- Boogard angle (Fig. 5.6): Formed by the intersection of McRae line and Wackenheim line. The normal angle is 126° ± 6°. If the angle measures more than 136°, it is indicative of platybasia.

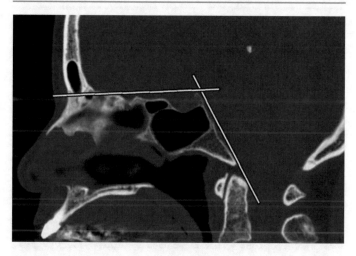

Fig. 5.5 Sagittal computed tomography (CT) image shows the basal angle

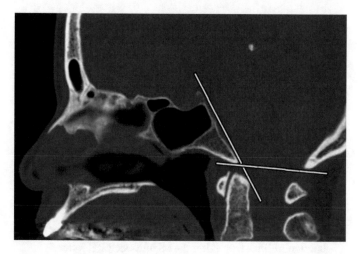

Fig. 5.6 Sagittal computed tomography (CT) image shows the Boogard angle

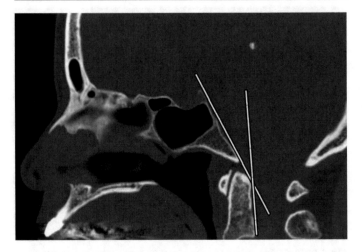

Fig. 5.7 Sagittal computed tomography (CT) image shows the clivoaxial angle

- Clivoaxial angle (Fig. 5.7): Formed by the intersection of the Wackenheim clivus baseline with a line drawn along the posterior surface of the axis body and odontoid process; it is a practical indicator for basilar invagination with high diagnostic value.

- Clivus canal angle (Fig. 5.8): The angle between the line extending from the top of the dorsum sellae to the basion and the line between the inferodorsal portions of C2 and the most superodorsal part of the dens. The angle normally varies from 150° in flexion to 180° in extension. An angle of less than 150° may be associated with ventral cord compression.

- Atlanto-occipital joint axis angle (Fig. 5.9): Formed at the junction of lines traversing the atlanto-occipital joints.
  - Average = 124°–127°
  - May approach 180° in severe occipital condyle hypoplasia

- Atlanto-occipital interval (Fig. 5.10): Distance between the posterior aspect of the anterior arch of the atlas and the dens.

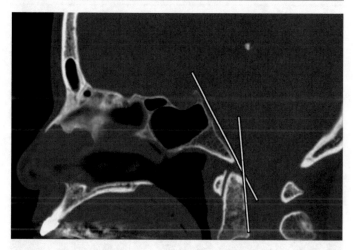

Fig. 5.8 Sagittal computed tomography (CT) image shows the clivus canal angle

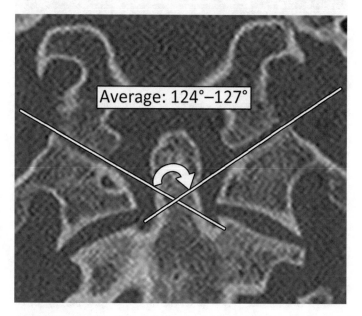

Fig. 5.9 Coronal computed tomography (CT) image shows the atlanto-occipital joint axis angle

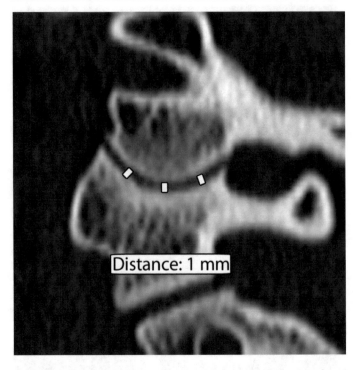

Distance: 1 mm

Fig. 5.10 Sagittal computed tomography (CT) image shows the atlanto-occipital interval

The mean value is 1.0 mm (95% of adults measure between 0.6 and 1.4 mm and 97.5% of children measure less than 2.5 mm at any point along the joint space).

- Basion-dens interval (Fig. 5.11): Shortest distance between the most inferior aspect of the basion and the nearest ossified point of the superior aspect of the dens in the midsagittal plane. If an os odontoideum is present, the measurement extends from the basion to the top of the os odontoideum. Widening can be a sign of craniovertebral junction injury, with a maximum of 9 mm in adults. In children, the basion-cartilaginous dens

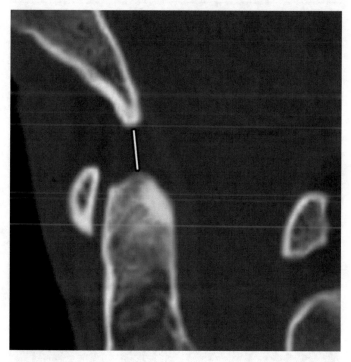

Fig. 5.11 Sagittal computed tomography (CT) image shows the basion-dens interval

interval is the counterpart that can be used with upper limits as follows:
- Ages 0–3 years: 5.3 mm
- Ages 3–6 years: 5.6 mm
- Ages 6–10 years: 7.2 mm

• Basion-axial interval (Fig. 5.12): Distance between the basion and the superior extension of the posterior cortical margin of the dens in the midsagittal plane. This measurement is normally less than 12 mm.

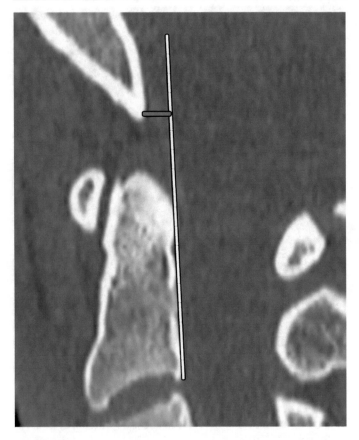

Fig. 5.12 Sagittal computed tomography (CT) image shows the basion-axial interval

- Atlanto-dens interval (Fig. 5.13): Line from the posterior aspect of the anterior arch of C1 to the most anterior aspect of the dens at the midpoint of the thickness of the arch in craniocaudal dimension; normal when less than 2 mm.

- The Powers ratio (Fig. 5.14): Calculated by dividing the distance from the tip of the basion to the midpoint of the anterior

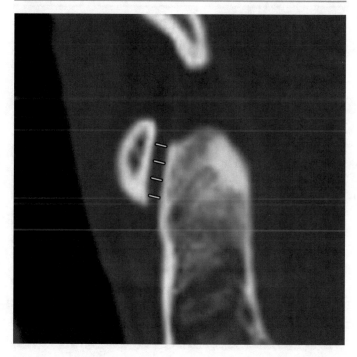

Fig. 5.13 Sagittal computed tomography (CT) image shows the atlanto-dens interval

aspect of the posterior arch of C1 by the distance from the tip of the opisthion to the midpoint of the posterior aspect of the anterior arch of C1 in the midline. It is used in the evaluation of atlanto-occipital dissociation and is considered normal when less than 1.

Practical Implications
- Congenital and acquired conditions that can manifest with abnormal craniocervical junction measurements include rheumatoid arthritis, osteomalacia, Paget disease, Chiari malformation, Klippel-Feil and Down syndromes, achondroplasia, mucopolysaccharidoses, osteogenesis imperfecta, as well as trauma.

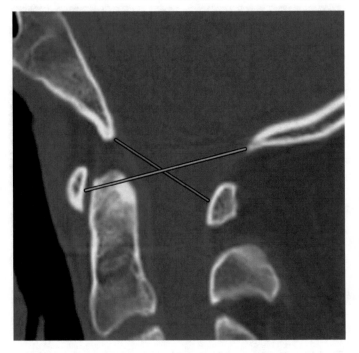

Fig. 5.14 Sagittal computed tomography (CT) image shows the lines between the tip of the basion to the midpoint of the anterior aspect of the posterior arch of C1 (red) and from the tip of the opisthion to the midpoint of the posterior aspect of the anterior arch of C1 (green) used to determine the Powers ratio

- Reference to craniocervical metrics is useful for identifying suspected cases of atlanto-axial separation (Fig. 5.15) and occipital-cervical dislocation (Fig. 5.16), which otherwise may not be accompanied by other abnormalities on CT, yet can be associated with a high rate of neurologic morbidity and mortality if undiagnosed.
- Basilar invagination refers to developmental anomalies of the craniovertebral junction in which the superior aspect of the odontoid extends above the foramen magnum, while basilar

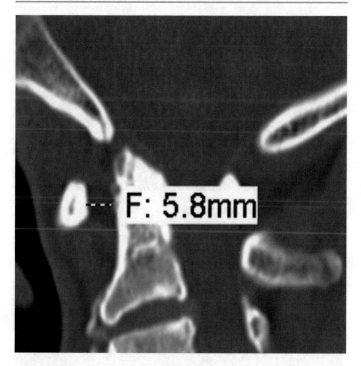

Fig. 5.15 Atlanto-axial separation. Sagittal computed tomography (CT) image shows widening of the atlanto-axial interval in a trauma patient

impression refers to acquired conditions of the craniovertebral junction in which the superior aspect of the odontoid extends above the foramen magnum (Fig. 5.17). This can be accompanied by compression of the spinal cord.
- Platybasia is flattening of the central skull base (Fig. 5.18). This can be accompanied by basilar invagination and other craniocervical junction abnormities. Given the altered anatomy, a transnasal approach may be preferable to a transcervical endoscopic approach for accessing the craniocervical junction in patients with platybasia.

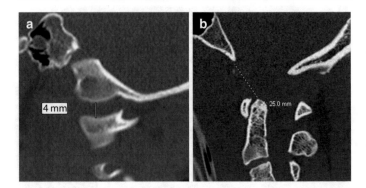

Fig. 5.16 Atlanto-occipital dislocation. Sagittal computed tomography (CT) image shows wide separation between the occipital condyle and lateral mass of C1 in a pediatric trauma patient (**a**) and widening of the basion-dens interval in an adult (**b**)

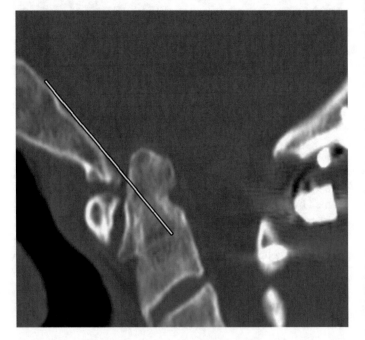

Fig. 5.17 Basilar invagination. Sagittal computed tomography (CT) image shows marked extension of the dens above the foramen magnum, well beyond the Wackenheim clivus line, in a patient with rheumatoid arthritis

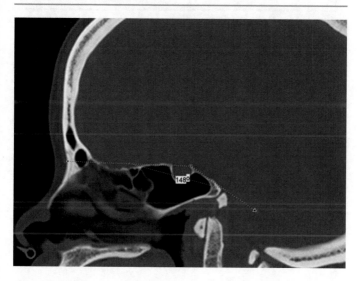

Fig. 5.18 Platybasia. Sagittal computed tomography (CT) image shows an obtuse basal angle and clival hypoplasia

Further Reading

Batista UC, Joaquim AF, Fernandes YB, Mathias RN, Ghizoni E, Tedeschi H. Computed tomography evaluation of the normal craniocervical junction craniometry in 100 asymptomatic patients. Neurosurg Focus. 2015;38(4):E5.

Bertozzi JC, Rojas CA, Martinez CR. Evaluation of the pediatric craniocervical junction on MDCT. AJR Am J Roentgenol. 2009;192(1):26–31.

Botelho RV, Ferreira ED. Angular craniometry in craniocervical junction malformation. Neurosurg Rev. 2013;36(4):603–10; discussion 610.

El-Sayed IH, Wu JC, Dhillon N, Ames CP, Mummaneni P. The importance of platybasia and the palatine line in patient selection for endonasal surgery of the craniocervical junction: a radiographic study of 12 patients. World Neurosurg. 2011;76(1–2):183–8; discussion 74–8.

Ji W, Wang XY, Xu HZ, Yang XD, Chi YL, Yang JS, Yan SF, Zheng JW, Chen ZX. The anatomic study of clival screw fixation for the craniovertebral region. Eur Spine J. 2012;21(8):1483–91.

Koenigsberg RA, Vakil N, Hong TA, Htaik T, Faerber E, Maiorano T, Dua M, Faro S, Gonzales C. Evaluation of platybasia with MR imaging. AJNR Am J Neuroradiol. 2005;26(1):89–92.

Rojas CA, Bertozzi JC, Martinez CR, Whitlow J. Reassessment of the cranio-cervical junction: normal values on CT. AJNR Am J Neuroradiol. 2007;28(9):1819–23. Epub 2007 Sep 24.

Singh AK, Fulton Z, Tiwari R, Zhang X, Lu L, Altmeyer WB, Tantiwongkosi B. Basion-cartilaginous dens interval: an imaging parameter for cranio-vertebral junction assessment in children. AJNR Am J Neuroradiol. 2017;38(12):2380–4.

Xu S, Gong R. Clivodens angle: a new diagnostic method for basilar invagi-nation at computed tomography. Spine (Phila Pa 1976). 2016a;41(17):1365–71.

Xu S, Gong R. Clivus height value: a new diagnostic method for basilar invagination at CT. Clin Radiol. 2016b;71(11):1200.e1–5.

Normative Measurements of Head and Neck Lymph Nodes on Imaging

6

Grayson W. Hooper and
Daniel Thomas Ginat

6.1 Imaging Modalities

6.1.1 Computed Tomography (CT)

- CT soft tissue images with 1–3 mm section thickness can be used to accurately determine the location, size, and gross morphology of head and neck lymph nodes.
- Normal lymph nodes have attenuation similar to that of muscle.
- Intravenous contrast administration can help with characterization of lymph node consistency, such as the presence of necrosis.

G. W. Hooper
Department of Radiology, Fort Belvoir Community Hospital,
Fort Belvoir, VA, USA

D. T. Ginat (✉)
Department of Radiology, Section of Neuroradiology, University of
Chicago, Chicago, IL, USA
e-mail: dtg1@uchicago.edu

© Springer Nature Switzerland AG 2021
D. T. Ginat (ed.), *Manual of Normative Measurements in Head
and Neck Imaging*, https://doi.org/10.1007/978-3-030-50567-7_6

6.1.2   Magnetic Resonance Imaging (MRI)

- Normal lymph nodes display homogeneous T1 and T2 signal and enhancement.
- The optimal contrast between abnormal lymph nodes and muscle is achieved using a long repetition time (TR) and a long echo time (TE), although greater signal-to-noise ratio in MRI is achieved using a long TR and a short TE.
- Diffusion-weighted imaging (DWI) can be helpful in detecting subcentimeter metastatic lymph nodes in the setting of head and neck cancer, in which metastatic cervical lymph nodes generally have lower diffusivity as compared with benign lymph nodes.
- MRI contrast resolution is superior to that of CT and therefore is more sensitive for the detection of extracapsular spread than CT, as well as for discerning retropharyngeal lymph nodes, but MRI is generally not as reliable as CT for delineating lower neck lymph nodes due to the frequent presence of artifacts.

6.1.3   Ultrasound

- Ultrasound is used adjunctively in the evaluation of head and neck neoplasms and nodal metastasis.
- Ultrasound has the advantage of dynamic real time soft tissue evaluation, which can show detailed lymph node characteristics.
- Ultrasound has been shown to have both higher sensitivity and specificity for nodal metastasis when compared to CT.
- Ultrasound is limited in evaluating the deep lymph nodes of the neck. It is also user dependent, which contributes to imaging variability.

- The addition of ultrasound to CT can spare patients secondary surgery after sentinel node biopsy.

6.1.4 ^{18}Fluoro-2-Deoxy-D-Glucose Positron Emission Tomography (^{18}FDG-PET)

- ^{18}FDG-PET provides an assessment of soft tissue metabolism through standardized uptake values (SUV) and has a higher sensitivity and specificity than CT for the detection of lymph node metastases in patients with head and neck cancer, but is routinely combined with CT or MRI for greater anatomic delineation.
- A lymph node SUVmax/liver SUVmax ratio ≥0.90 can be used as a threshold for detecting cervical metastatic nodes with an accuracy of 90%.
- ^{18}FDG-PET can reliably detect metastatic neck lymph nodes that measure ≥10 mm, but intranodal tumor or metastatic lymph nodes smaller than 5 mm are generally not detectable.
- Regardless of size, certain cancers tend not to be FDG avid, such as adenoid cystic carcinomas.

6.2 RECIST Criteria

The response evaluation criteria in solid tumors (RECIST) was created in 2000 and updated in 2009 as a means of objectively measuring solid tumor response to therapy. Updated guidelines (RECIST 1.1) measure the longest dimension of the target lesion and the shortest dimension of lymph nodes in the axial plane with a minimum threshold of 15 mm. This measurement strategy also pertains to the most recent iRECIST guidelines for immunotherapy response. The short axis is determined by first identifying the long axis or the longest diameter of a lymph node and then measuring

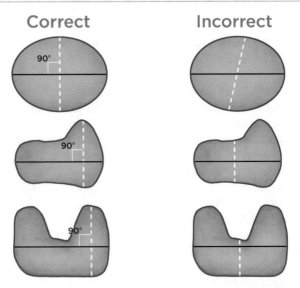

Fig. 6.1 Illustration depicting correct and incorrect approaches for measuring lymph nodes

the widest perpendicular diameter (Fig. 6.1). Similarly, if abnormal lymph nodes have coalesced such that they are no longer separable, the vector of the longest diameter of the overall lesion should be used to determine the perpendicular vector for the maximal short-axis diameter of the coalesced lesion (Fig. 6.2). Coalescent lymphadenopathy is an independent risk factor for poor prognosis in the setting of oropharyngeal squamous cell carcinoma.

6.3   Lymph Node Stations

6.3.1   Cervical Lymph Nodes

The cervical lymph node levels are delineated by recognizable anatomic landmarks, as illustrated in Fig. 6.3.

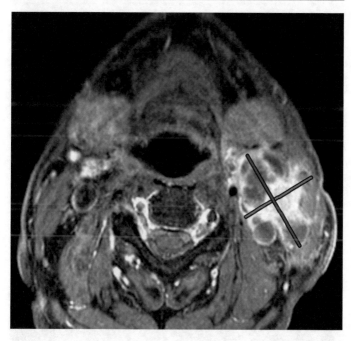

Fig. 6.2 Axial post-contrast T1-weighted magnetic resonance imaging (MRI) image shows a conglomerate of necrotic left cervical lymph node metastases with long axis (blue line) and short axis (red line) dimensions

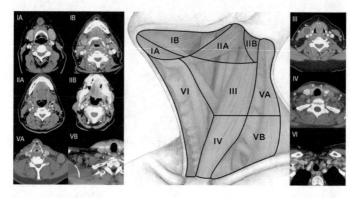

Fig. 6.3 Diagram of the cervical lymph node levels

If the short axis exceeds 11 mm in the jugulodigastric region and 10 mm in all other lateral compartment cervical nodes, and 8 mm for central compartment lymph nodes, metastasis is probably present in adults. The normal maximum long-axis size of jugulodigastric nodes in cancer patients is 15 mm. However, level 2 lymph nodes can normally measure up to 15 mm or more in children (Fig. 6.4). In addition, a ratio between the long- and short-axis diameters of less than 1.5, or a rounded lymph node, is suggestive of metastatic disease. Nevertheless, there is an error rate of 10–20% based on size criteria alone. Ultimately, there is a tradeoff between sensitivity and specify for size thresholds. Indeed, up to 50% of lymph nodes measuring less than 5 mm har-

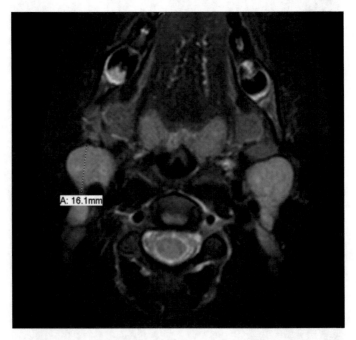

Fig. 6.4 Normal cervical lymph nodes in a child. Axial T2-weighted magnetic resonance imaging (MRI) shows plump cervical lymph nodes bilaterally along with tonsillar tissues in a 3-year-old infant without lymph node disease

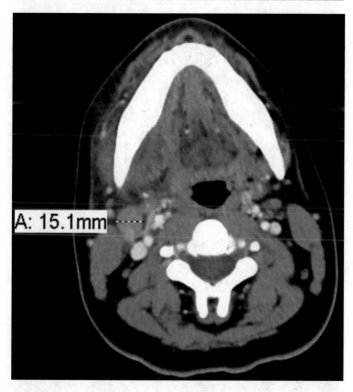

A: 15.1mm

Fig. 6.5 Reactive lymph node. Axial computed tomography (CT) image shows an enlarged right level 2 lymph node associated with right mandibular odontogenic infection

bor micrometastases that are occult on imaging. Alternatively, lymph node enlargement can result from benign inflammatory or reactive processes (Fig. 6.5).

Other features to consider besides size on imaging include the presence of cystic or necrotic components and effacement of the fatty hilum (Fig. 6.6). [18]FDG-PET can sometimes be helpful in detecting hypermetabolic metastatic lymphadenopathy that is smaller than size criteria. The presence of calcifications can also be a sign of metastatic disease, particularly in the setting of thyroid cancer (Fig. 6.7). Extracapsular spread is another feature of

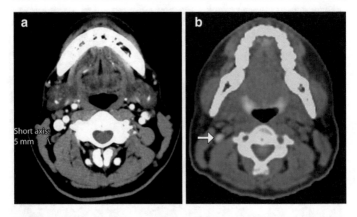

Fig. 6.6 Necrotic lymph node. Axial computed tomography (CT) image (**a**) shows a small right level 2B lymph node with a hypoattenuating area in a patient with nasopharyngeal carcinoma, which proved to be metastatic disease. The corresponding [18]FDG-PET/CT image (**b**) shows the small lymph node is hypermetabolic (arrow)

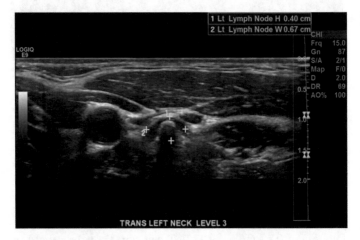

Fig. 6.7 Lymph node with calcification from metastatic thyroid cancer. Gray-scale ultrasound image shows the calcification with shadowing within a small level 3 lymph node

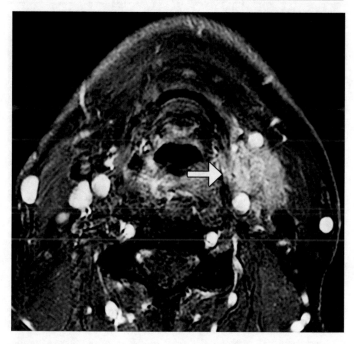

Fig. 6.8 Extracapsular spread. Axial post-contrast T1-weighted magnetic resonance imaging (MRI) shows a left cervical lymph node with infiltrative margins (arrow)

malignant lymphadenopathy that portends a relatively poor prognosis and is characterized by the presence of irregular margins and loss of adjacent fat planes, which is best delineated via MRI (Fig. 6.8). Furthermore, it is important to consider the presence of nodal grouping, which refers to three or more contiguous and confluent lymph nodes, each of which has a maximal diameter of 6–15 mm (Fig. 6.9). Such a grouping in the drainage chain of the tumor is suggestive of metastatic disease.

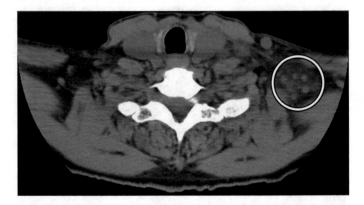

Fig. 6.9 Nodal grouping. Axial computed tomography (CT) image shows a cluster of left supraclavicular subcentimeter lymph nodes, which proved to be metastatic disease

Level I: Submental and Submandibular

- This nodal level is bounded by the mylohyoid muscle superiorly and the inferior margin of the hyoid inferiorly. It is further subdivided into sections "A" and "B" with level IA described as submental, between the anterior bellies of the digastric musculature. Level IB or submandibular lymph nodes are found posterolateral to the digastric muscles and anterior to the submandibular glands.
- The submental lymph nodes receive lymphatic drainage from:
  - Central inferior lip
  - Apex of the tongue
  - Floor of the mouth
- The submandibular lymph nodes receive lymphatic drainage from:
  - Facial lymph nodes
  - Cheeks
  - Lateral aspects of the nose
  - Oral cavity
  - Submental nodes
- Submandibular lymph nodes can assume a more rounded configuration (S/L > 0.5), which is different from the oval shape expected in other nodal stations (3).

Level II: Anterior Cervical/Upper Jugular

- This station is bounded superiorly by the base of the skull and inferiorly by the hyoid bone. It is bounded posteriorly by the posterior margin of the sternocleidomastoid and anteriorly by the posterior margin of the submandibular glands. Level II lymph nodes can be further subdivided into IIA and IIB. Level IIA lymph nodes are located posterior or otherwise tangent to the internal jugular vein. Level IIB lymph nodes are located posterior to the internal jugular vein and are separated from it by a fat plane.
- Level II lymph nodes receive lymphatic drainage from:
  - Oropharynx
  - Posterior aspect of the mouth
  - Parotid glands

Level III: Middle Jugular

- These lymph nodes are bounded superiorly by the inferior margin of the hyoid and inferiorly by the superior margin of the cricoid cartilage. The posterior boundary is posterior margin of the sternocleidomastoid muscle.
- The lymph nodes of this station receive lymphatic drainage from:
  - Larynx
  - Hypopharynx

Level IV: Inferior Jugular

- The inferior jugular lymph nodes are demarcated superiorly by the inferior margin of the cricoid cartilage and inferiorly by the superior surface of the clavicle. They are bounded anteriorly by the internal or common carotid artery, which separates level IV from level VI lymph nodes.
- Level IV lymph nodes receive lymphatic drainage from:
  - Subglottic soft tissues
  - Thyroid
  - Cervical esophagus

Level V: Spinal Accessory/Posterior Triangle

- These lymph nodes are posterior to the sternocleidomastoid muscle posterior margin and anterior to the anterior margin of the trapezius. They are arranged from cranial to caudal with the superior margin being the skull base and the inferior margin being the superior cortical surface of the clavicle. They can further be divided into VA above the cricoid and VB below the cricoid.
- Level V lymph nodes receive lymphatic drainage from:
  - Nasopharynx
  - Posterior neck
  - Posterior scalp

Level VI: Visceral

- The visceral lymph nodes are bounded by the hyoid bone superiorly and the medial aspects of the internal carotid arteries bilaterally.
- Level VI lymph nodes receive lymphatic drainage from:
  - Cervical esophagus
  - Thyroid
  - Larynx

6.3.2 Retropharyngeal Lymph Nodes

- Retropharyngeal lymph nodes are located anterior to the alar fascia at the level of the C1 vertebra and consist of medial and lateral lymph nodes.
- A short-axis diameter cutoff of 5–6 mm has been recommended as the size criterion for metastatic lateral retropharyngeal lymph nodes in adults or any node with central necrosis (Fig. 6.10).
- Retropharyngeal lymph nodes are larger in children than in adults. In particular, the mean size of lateral retropharyngeal lymph nodes is 7 mm in young children (Fig. 6.11), but these lymph nodes significantly shrink after 5 years of age.

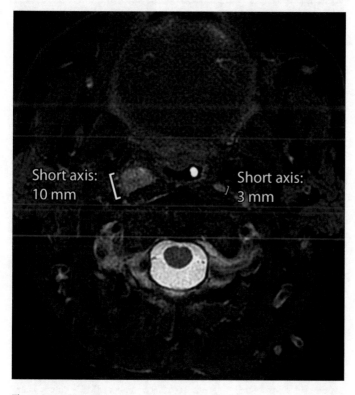

Fig. 6.10 Retropharyngeal lymphadenopathy. Axial fat-suppressed T2-weighted magnetic resonance imaging (MRI) shows a metastatic right lateral retropharyngeal lymph node that measures 10 mm in short axis and a normal left lateral retropharyngeal lymph node

- The medial retropharyngeal lymph nodes regress by adulthood.
- Retropharyngeal lymph nodes receive drainage from:
  - Nasal cavity
  - Paranasal sinuses
  - Upper pharynx
  - Oral cavity
  - Middle ear

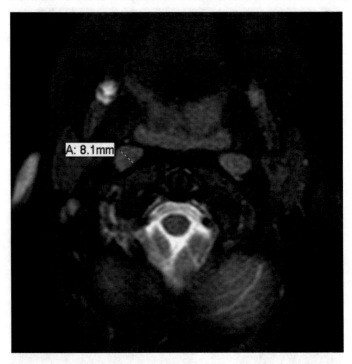

Fig. 6.11 Normal pediatric retropharyngeal lymph node. Axial fat-suppressed T2-weighted magnetic resonance imaging (MRI) shows lateral retropharyngeal lymph nodes that measure up to 8 mm in short axis

6.3.3 Parotid Lymph Nodes

- Parotid lymph nodes are comprised of superficial, extrafascial, subfascial extraglandular, and deep intraglandular nodes.
- The superficial extrafascial parotid lymph nodes are superficial to the superficial layer of the deep cervical fascia.
- The subfascial extraglandular group lymph nodes are deep to the fascia, but not in the parotid glandular tissue.
- The deep intraglandular lymph nodes are located within the parotid gland tissues, usually lateral to the retromandibular vein.

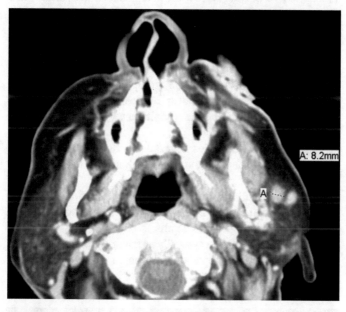

Fig. 6.12 Parotid lymphadenopathy. Axial computed tomography (CT) image shows a left face cutaneous squamous cell carcinoma with enlarged left parotid lymph nodes

- The average volume of normal parotid lymph nodes is 0.1 mL.
- A cutoff of 5 mm for the short axis of parotid lymph nodes has been proposed (Fig. 6.12).
- The parotid lymph nodes receive lymphatic drainage from:
    - Face and anterior scalp
    - Eyelids
    - Auricle and external auditory
    - Tympanic membrane and part of the Eustachian tube
    - Superficial preauricular lymph nodes
    - Posterior part of cheek
    - Parotid gland
    - Lacrimal glands

6.3.4   Occipital Lymph Nodes

- The occipital lymph nodes comprise the suprafascial, subfascial, and deep occipital node groups.
- The suprafascial or superficial group is intimately applied to the superficial layer of the deep cervical fascia or to the epicranial aponeurosis, along the occipital artery and great occipital nerve.
- The subfascial group lies near the superior nuchal line of the occipital bone, beneath the superficial layer of the deep cervical fascia.
- The deep occipital group lies beneath the superior insertion of splenius capitis, above the obliquus capitis superior, and medial to the longissimus capitis.
- Normal occipital nodes typically measure up to about 3–6 mm.
- Occipital lymphadenopathy can have an elongated morphology against the occipital bone (Fig. 6.13).

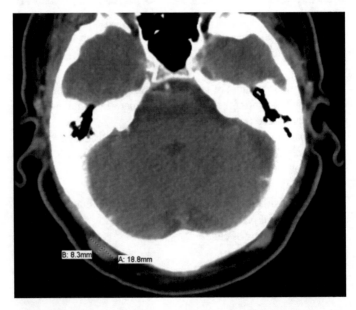

Fig. 6.13 Occipital lymphadenopathy. Axial computed tomography (CT) image shows enlarged lymph nodes in a patient with lymphoma

- Occipital nodes receive lymphatic drainage from:
  - Posterior part of the scalp
  - Posterior part of the upper neck

Further Reading

Ahuja AT, Ying M. Sonographic evaluation of cervical lymph nodes. Am J Roentgenol. 2005;184:1691–9.

Braams JW, Pruim J, Freling NJM, Nikkels PGJ, Boering G, et al. Detection of lymph node metastases of squamous-cell cancer of the head and neck with FDG-PET and MRI. J Nucl Med. 1995;36(2):211–6.

Chong V. Cervical lymphadenopathy: what radiologists need to know. Cancer Imaging. 2004;4(2):116–20.

Chung MS, Choi YJ, Kim SO, Lee YS, Hong JY, Lee JH, Baek JH. A scoring system for prediction of cervical lymph node metastasis in patients with head and neck squamous cell carcinoma. AJNR Am J Neuroradiol. 2019;40(6):1049–54.

Costa NS, Salisbury SR, Donnelly LF. Retropharyngeal lymph nodes in children: a common imaging finding and potential source of misinterpretation. AJR Am J Roentgenol. 2011;196(4):W433–7.

Costa E, Silva Souza LMB, Leung KJ, O'Neill A, Jayender J, Lee TC. Jugulodigastric lymph node size by age on CT in an adult cancer-free population. Clin Imaging. 2018;47:30–3.

Curtin HD, Ishwaran H, Mancuso AA, Dalley RW, Caudry DJ, McNeil BJ. Comparison of CT and MR imaging in staging of neck metastases. Radiology. 1998;207:123–30.

Dooms GC, Hricak H, Crooks LE, Higgins CB. Magnetic resonance imaging of the lymph nodes: comparison with CT. Radiology. 1984;153(3):719–28.

Eisenmenger LB, Wiggins RH III. Imaging of head and neck lymph nodes. Radiol Clin North Am. 2015;53(1):115–32.

Lengelé B, Hamoir M, Scalliet P, Grégoire V. Anatomical bases for the radiological delineation of lymph node areas. Major collecting trunks, head and neck. Radiother Oncol. 2007;85(1):146–55.

Leticia MB, Souza CS, Leung KJ, O'Neill A, Jagadeesan J, Lee TC. Jugulodigastric lymph node size by age on CT in an adult cancer-free population. Clin Imaging. 2018;47:30–3.

Lim RS, Ramdave S, Beech P, Billah B, Karim MN, Smith JA, Safdar A, Sigston E. Utility of SUVmax on 18 F-FDG PET in detecting cervical nodal metastases. Cancer Imaging. 2016;16(1):39.

Maeda T, Yamamoto Y, Furukawa H, Oyama A, Funayama E, Murao N, Hayashi T. Dominant lymph drainage patterns in the occipital and parietal regions: evaluation of lymph nodes in patients with skin cancer of the head. Int J Clin Oncol. 2017;22(4):774–9.

Nishio N, Fujimoto Y, Hiramatsu M, Maruo T, Tsuzuki H, Mukoyama N, Yokoi S, Wada A, Kaneko Furukawa M, Furukawa M, Sone M. Diagnosis of cervical lymph node metastases in head and neck cancer with ultrasonic measurement of lymph node volume. Auris Nasus Larynx. 46(6):889–95. pii: S0385-8146(18)30489-9.

Norling R, Buron BMD, Therkildsen MH, Henriksen BM, von Buchwald C, Nielsen MB. Staging of cervical lymph nodes in oral squamous cell carcinoma: adding ultrasound in clinically lymph node negative patients may improve diagnostic work-up. PLoS One. 2014;9:e90360.

Sathyanarayan V, Bharani S. Enlarged lymph nodes in head and neck cancer: analysis with triplex ultrasonography. Ann Maxillofac Surg. 2013;3(1):35–9.

Seymour L, Bogaerts J, Perrone A, Ford R, Schwartz LH, et al. iRECIST: guidelines for response criteria for use in trials testing immunotherapeutics. Lancet Oncol. 2017;18:e143–52.

Shetty SK, Harisinghani MD. Magnetic resonance techniques in lymph node imaging. Appl Radiol. 2004; accessed online. https://appliedradiology.com/articles/magnetic-resonance-techniques-in-lymph-node-imaging.

Som PM. Detection of metastasis in cervical lymph nodes: CT and MR criteria and differential diagnosis. AJR Am J Roentgenol. 1992;158(5):961–9.

Spector ME, Gallagher KK, Light E, Ibrahim M, Chanowski EJ, et al. Matted nodes: poor prognostic marker in oropharyngeal squamous cell carcinoma independent of HPV and EGFR status. Head Neck. 2012;34(12):1727–33.

Sun J, Li B, Li CJ, Li Y, Su F, Gao QH, et al. Computed tomography versus magnetic resonance imaging for diagnosing cervical lymph node metastasis of head and neck cancer: a systematic review and meta-analysis. Onco Targets Ther. 2015;8:1291–313.

Van den Brekel MWM, Stel HV, Castelijns JA, Nauta JJP, van der Waal I. Cervical lymph node metastasis: assessment of radiologic criteria. Radiology. 1990;177:379–84.

Van den Brekel MWM, Castelijns JA, Snow GB. The size of lymph nodes in the neck on sonograms as a radiologic criterion for metastasis: how reliable is it? AJNR Am J Neuroradiol. 1998;19:695–700.

Vandecaveye V, de Keyzer V, Dirix P, Verbeken E, Nuyts S, Hermans R. Head and neck squamous cell carcinoma: value of diffusion-weighted MR imaging for nodal staging. Radiology. 2009;251:134–46.

Veenstra HJ, Klop WM, Lohuis PJ, Nieweg OE, van Velthuysen ML, Balm AJ. Cadaver study on the location of suboccipital lymph nodes: guidance for suboccipital node dissection. Head Neck. 2014;36(5):682–6.

Ying M, Ahuja A, Brook F, Brown B, Metreweli C. Sonographic appearance and distribution of normal cervical lymph nodes in a Chinese population. J Ultrasound Med. 1996;15(6):431–6.

Ying M, Ahuja A, Brook F. Sonographic appearances of cervical lymph nodes: variations by age and sex. J Clin Ultrasound. 2002;30(1):1–11.

Zhang GY, Liu LZ, Wei WH, Deng YM, Li YZ, Liu XW. Radiologic criteria of retropharyngeal lymph node metastasis in nasopharyngeal carcinoma treated with radiation therapy. Radiology. 2010;255(2):605–12.

Zhang MH, Ginat DT. Normative measurements of parotid lymph nodes on CT imaging [published online ahead of print, 2020 May 14]. Surg Radiol Anat. 2020;10.1007/s00276-020-02494-8. https://doi.org/10.1007/s00276-020-02494-8.

Normative Measurements of the Thyroid, Salivary Glands, and Tonsils on Imaging

7

Daniel Thomas Ginat

7.1 Thyroid Gland

- The thyroid gland is located in the visceral space of the neck and consists of two lobes connected by an isthmus anterior to the trachea.
- The thyroid gland has a high iodine content, resulting in high attenuation of 80–100 Hounsfield unit (HU) on non-contrast computed tomography (CT) and an attenuation of 150–170 HU on post-contrast CT (Fig. 7.1).
- The normal dimensions of the thyroid in adults are 40–60 mm in craniocaudal and 13–18 mm in anteroposterior dimensions (Fig. 7.2).
- The mean thyroid volume in adults is 10.7 ± 2.8 mL (range: 5.7–17.1 mL) and the volume correlates with body size.
- The normal dimensions of thyroid gland in adult and pediatric groups are detailed in Tables 7.1 and 7.2.

D. T. Ginat (✉)
Department of Radiology, Section of Neuroradiology,
University of Chicago, Chicago, IL, USA
e-mail: dtg1@uchicago.edu

© Springer Nature Switzerland AG 2021
D. T. Ginat (ed.), *Manual of Normative Measurements in Head and Neck Imaging*, https://doi.org/10.1007/978-3-030-50567-7_7

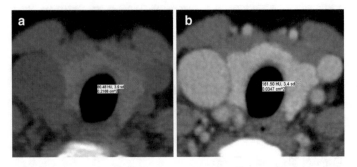

Fig. 7.1 Axial computed tomography (CT) images without (**a**) and with (**b**) contrast show the normally hyperattenuating and enhancing thyroid tissue

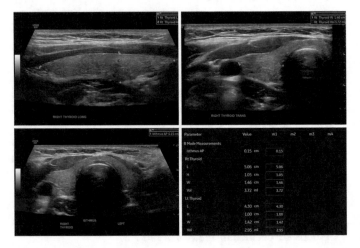

Fig. 7.2 Normal thyroid gland. Ultrasound images and Tables 7.1 and 7.2 show the dimensions of the thyroid gland and its components

- The pyramidal lobe is a remnant of the thyroglossal duct and is a superior extension of normal thyroid tissue. Its presence is relevant for thyroid cancer surgery.
- The mean anteroposterior diameter, transverse diameter, and length of the pyramidal lobe are 2, 6, and 21 mm, respectively (Fig. 7.3).

Table 7.1 Thyroid measurements in adults

Morphologic parameter	Size
Anteroposterior length, right (mm)	13.5 ± 2.0
Anteroposterior length, left (mm)	13.1 ± 1.8
Transverse length, right (mm)	16.0 ± 3.0
Transverse length, left (mm)	15.3 ± 2.5
Longitudinal length, right (mm)	42.5 ± 4.9
Longitudinal length, left (mm)	40.2 ± 3.8
Isthmus thickness (mm)	2.5 ± 1.0
Volume, right (cm³)	4.6 ± 2.0
Volume, left (cm³)	4.0 ± 1.4
Volume, total (cm³)	8.6 ± 3.1

Table 7.2 Pediatric thyroid volumes by age

Age	Volume (cm³)
6	1.8 ± 0.4
8	1.8 ± 0.4
10	1.9 ± 0.5
12	2.8 ± 0.7
14	3.7 ± 0.7
16	5.0 ± 1.5

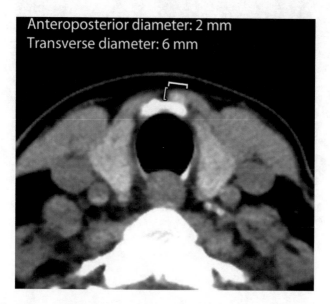

Anteroposterior diameter: 2 mm
Transverse diameter: 6 mm

Fig. 7.3 Pyramidal lobe. Axial computed tomography (CT) image shows the dimensions of the pyramidal lobe

7.1.1   Practical Implications

- Imaging can be obtained to evaluate patients with goiter and associated thyroid nodules, substernal extension, and tracheal narrowing (Fig. 7.4).
- When the longitudinal length of the lobes and the width of the whole gland together measure 6.5 cm or more, the thyroid gland can be considered enlarged.

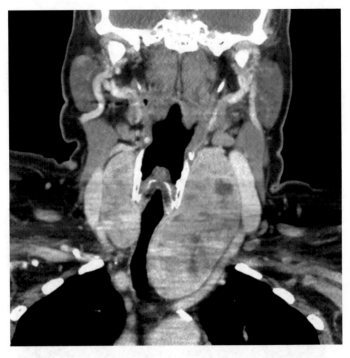

Fig. 7.4 Coronal computed tomography (CT) image shows goiter with tracheal narrowing

7.2   Parotid Gland and Ducts

- The parotid glands have a lobular morphology and can be divided into deep and superficial lobes, as well as an inferior projection referred to as the "tail," which can be defined as the inferior 2 cm of the gland.
- Based on CT or magnetic resonance imaging (MRI), the maximum axial width can range from 26 to 67 mm; the depth can range from 33 to 86 mm; and the height can range from 38 to 80 mm (Fig. 7.5).

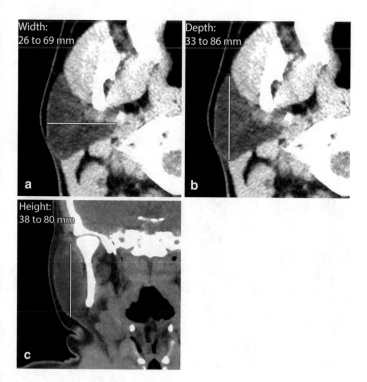

Fig. 7.5 Axial (**a** and **b**) and coronal (**c**) computed tomography (CT) images with the range of normal dimensions of the parotid gland

- Based on ultrasound, the parotid glands measure 46 ± 8 mm in the axis parallel to the mandibular ramus and 37 ± 6 mm in a transverse axis.
- The volumes of parotid glands among different demographic groups are listed in Table 7.3.
- Besides the actual size of the parotid gland, it can be helpful to consider symmetry of the glands, in which the glands typically measure within 10% on either side.
- The attenuation of the parotid glands normally decreases with age as the gland undergoes fatty infiltration (Fig. 7.6).

Table 7.3 Normal parotid gland volume

Demographic group	Volume (cm³)
Adolescent males	17–21
Adolescent females	14–17
Young adult males	20–24
Young adult females	18–21
Middle-aged males	29–35
Middle-aged females	20–22
Elderly males	29–35
Elderly females	29–35

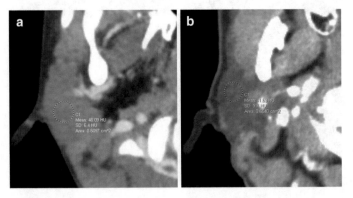

Fig. 7.6 Axial computed tomography (CT) images show higher attenuation of the parotid gland in a child (**a**) than in an adult (**b**)

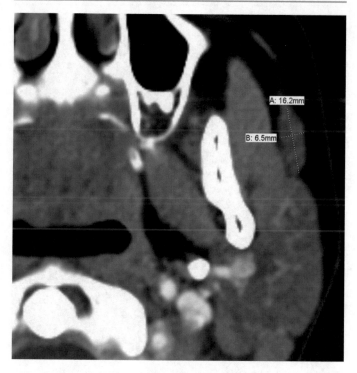

Fig. 7.7 Axial computed tomography (CT) image shows an accessory parotid gland

- The mean size of the accessory parotid gland is 16 mm × 6 mm and the mean distance from the main parotid gland is 10 mm (Fig. 7.7).
- The mean parotid duct length is 50 mm.
- The mean width of the parotid duct is normally 1–2 mm (Fig. 7.8).

7.2.1 Practical Implications

- Enlargement of the parotid gland can be due to sialosis, infectious and inflammatory sialadenitis, and neoplasm

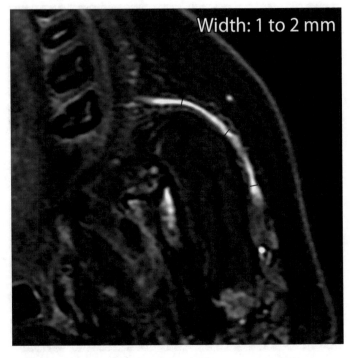

Fig. 7.8 Axial T2-weighted magnetic resonance imaging (MRI) shows a normal fluid-filled parotid duct

(Fig. 7.9). Some of these conditions can also be associated with parotid ductal dilatation (Fig. 7.10).

- A small parotid gland can result from post-inflammatory atrophy or can appear reduced in size after partial parotidectomy (Fig. 7.11).

7.3 Submandibular Gland and Ducts

- The normal submandibular gland measures 28 × 18 mm (±5 mm) in the axial plane (Fig. 7.12).
- The volume of submandibular glands in different demographic groups are listed in Table 7.4.

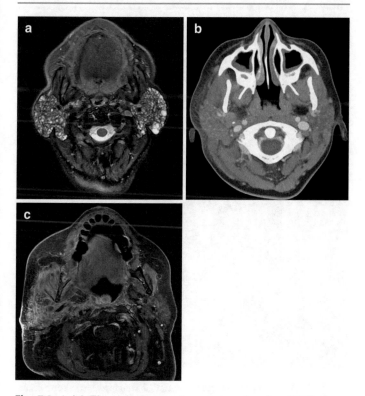

Fig. 7.9 Axial T2-weighted magnetic resonance imaging (MRI) shows enlarged parotid glands with multiple cysts related to Sjogren syndrome (**a**). Axial computed tomography (CT) image shows right parotid swelling related to parotitis with surrounding inflammation (**b**). Axial fat-suppressed post-contrast T1-weighted MRI shows diffuse infiltration of the right parotid gland from carcinoma (**c**)

- The mean length of the submandibular duct is 58 mm and the submandibular duct genu has a mean angle of 115° (Fig. 7.13).
- The mean width of the submandibular duct is 2–3 mm.
- An intra- or extra-glandular duct diameter of 3 mm or more indicates possible obstruction.

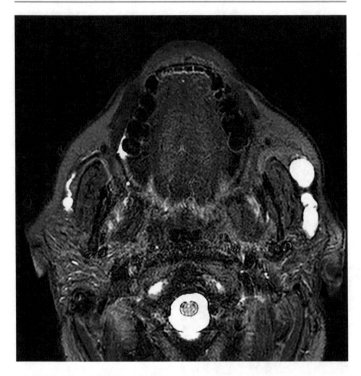

Fig. 7.10 Parotid ductal enlargment. Axial T2-weighted MRI shows dilatation of the bilateral parotid ducts, left greater than right, due to post-inflammatory strictures

7.3.1   Practical Implications

As with the parotid glands, the submandibular glands can be enlarged due to sialadenitis or neoplasm (Fig. 7.14). On the other hand, the glands can be small after radiation therapy or chronic inflammation (Fig. 7.15). Enlargement of the submandibular duct can be congenital due to an imperforate submandibular duct, or result from obstruction by tumors, post-inflammatory strictures, and calculi (Fig. 7.16).

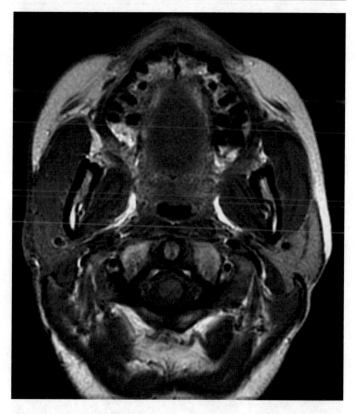

Fig. 7.11 Axial T1-weighted magnetic resonance imaging (MRI) shows a small amount of residual right parotid tissue following parotidectomy with scar tissue in the overlying subcutaneous tissues

7.4   Tonsils

- The tonsils comprise the lingual, palatine, and nasopharyngeal (adenoid) tonsils.
- The tonsils grow proportionally to the skeletal structures during childhood.

Table 7.4 Normal submandibular gland volume

Demographic group	Volume (cm³)
Adolescent males	7.2–8.9
Adolescent females	6.5–8.1
Young adult males	7.8–9.5
Young adult females	7.3–8.6
Middle-aged males	8.4–10.2
Middle-aged females	7.9–9.3
Elderly males	8.3–10.5
Elderly females	7.0–8.2

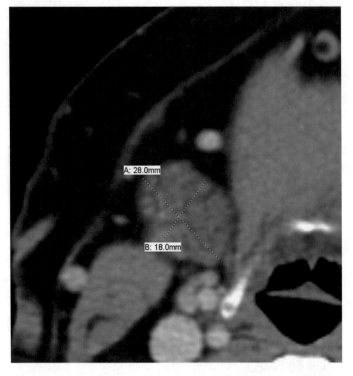

Fig. 7.12 Axial computed tomography (CT) image shows a normal submandibular gland

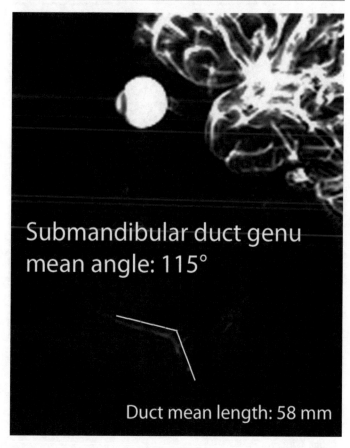

Fig. 7.13 Submandibular duct. Sagittal oblique magnetic resonance (MR) sialogram image shows the normal dimension of a normal submandibular duct

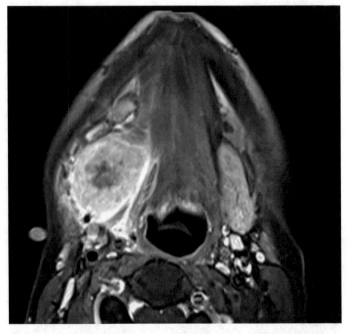

Fig. 7.14 Axial post-contrast T1-weighted MRI shows enlargement of the right submandibular gland due to an infiltrating carcinoma

- The adenoids are largest in the 7–10 years age group with a mean of 15 mm and steadily decline to 5 mm by 60 years of age (Fig. 7.17).
- The lingual tonsils typically measure less than 10 mm in thickness (Fig. 7.18).
- The normal adult palatine tonsils measure up to 12 mm × 20 mm in axial section (Fig. 7.19).

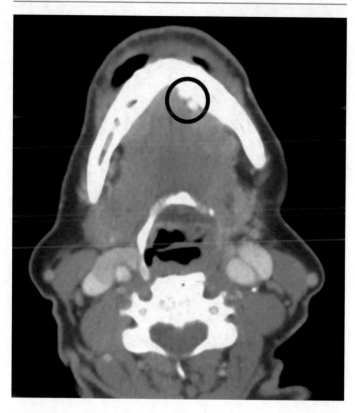

Fig. 7.15 Axial CT image shows atrophy of the left submandibular gland due to chronic sialadenitis from calculi (encircled)

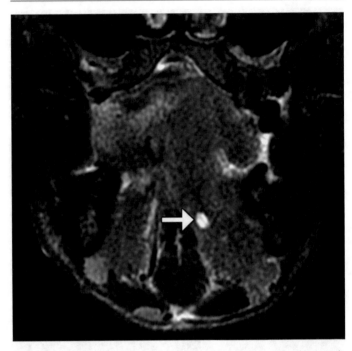

Fig. 7.16 Submandibular duct dilatation. Coronal T2-weighted magnetic resonance imaging (MRI) shows a dilated left submandibular duct (arrow) due to obstruction by tumor

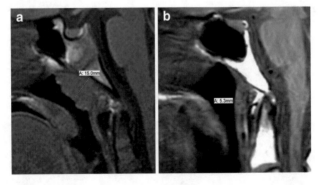

Fig. 7.17 Sagittal T1-weighted MR images in a child (**a**) and adult (**b**) show normal adenoids

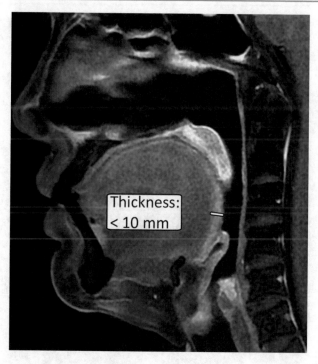

Fig. 7.18 Sagittal post-contrast T1-weighted magnetic resonance imaging (MRI) shows the normal lingual tonsils

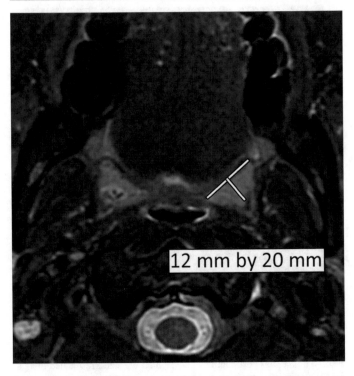

12 mm by 20 mm

Fig. 7.19 Axial fat-suppressed T2-weighted magnetic resonance imaging (MRI) shows normal palatine tonsils

7.4.1 Practical Implications

The tonsillar tissues can be enlarged due to benign lymphoid hyperplasia, infection, or neoplasm (Fig. 7.20).

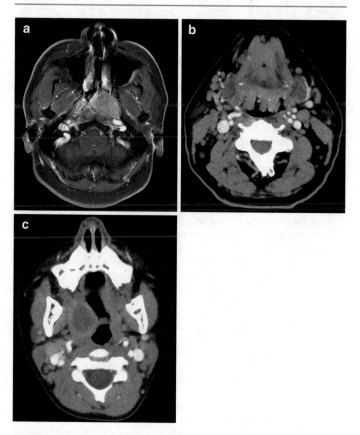

Fig. 7.20 Axial post-contrast T1-weighted magnetic resonance imaging (MRI) shows a nasopharyngeal carcinoma (**a**). Axial computed tomography (CT) image shows lingual tonsil hyperplasia (**b**). Axial CT image shows right tonsillitis with peritonsillar abscess (**c**)

Further Reading

Aasen S, Kolbenstvedt A. CT appearances of normal and obstructed submandibular duct. Acta Radiol. 1992;33(5):414–9.

Ahn D, Yeo CK, Han SY, Kim JK. The accessory parotid gland and facial process of the parotid gland on computed tomography. PLoS One. 2017;12(9):e0184633.

Atkinson C, Fuller J 3rd, Huang B. Cross-sectional imaging techniques and normal anatomy of the salivary glands. Neuroimaging Clin N Am. 2018;28(2):137–58.

Bhatia KS, King AD, Vlantis AC, Ahuja AT, Tse GM. Nasopharyngeal mucosa and adenoids: appearance at MR imaging. Radiology. 2012;263(2):437–43.

Ceylan I, Yener S, Bayraktar F, Secil M. Roles of ultrasound and power Doppler ultrasound for diagnosis of Hashimoto thyroiditis in anti-thyroid marker-positive euthyroid subjects. Quant Imaging Med Surg. 2014;4(4):232–8.

Dost P. Ultrasonographic biometry in normal salivary glands. Eur Arch Otorhinolaryngol. 1997;254(Suppl 1):S18–9.

Dost P, Kaiser S. Ultrasonographic biometry in salivary glands. Ultrasound Med Biol. 1997;23(9):1299–303.

Fricke BL, Donnelly LF, Shott SR, Kalra M, Poe SA, Chini BA, Amin RS. Comparison of lingual tonsil size as depicted on MR imaging between children with obstructive sleep apnea despite previous tonsillectomy and adenoidectomy and normal controls. Pediatr Radiol. 2006;36(6):518–23.

Friedman M, Wilson MN, Pulver TM, et al. Measurements of adult lingual tonsil tissue in health and disease. Otolaryngol Head Neck Surg. 2010;142(4):520–5.

Ginat DT. Imaging of benign neoplastic and nonneoplastic salivary gland tumors. Neuroimaging Clin N Am. 2018;28(2):159–69.

Hamilton BE, Salzman KL, Wiggins RH, Harnsberger HR. Earring lesions of the parotid tail. AJNR Am J Neuroradiol. 2003;24(9):1757–64.

Hong HS, Lee JY, Jeong SH. Normative values for tonsils in pediatric populations based on ultrasonography. J Ultrasound Med. 2018;37(7):1657–63.

Horsburgh A, Massoud TF. The salivary ducts of Wharton and Stenson: analysis of normal variant sialographic morphometry and a historical review. Ann Anat. 2013;195(3):238–42.

Ivanac G, Rozman B, Skreb F, Brkljacić B, Pavić L. Ultrasonographic measurement of the thyroid volume. Coll Antropol. 2004;28(1):287–91.

Kim DW, Jung SL, Baek JH, Kim J, Ryu JH, Na DG, Park SW, Kim JH, Sung JY, Lee Y, Rho MH. The prevalence and features of thyroid pyramidal lobe, accessory thyroid, and ectopic thyroid as assessed by computed tomography: a multicenter study. Thyroid. 2013;23(1):84–91.

Larsson SG, Lufkin RB, Hoover LA. Computed tomography of the subman-dibular salivary glands. Acta Radiol. 1987;28(6):693–6.

Li W, Sun ZP, Liu XJ, Yu GY. [Volume measurements of human parotid and submandibular glands]. Beijing Da Xue Xue Bao Yi Xue Ban. 2014;46(2):288–93.

Mahne A, El-Haddad G, Alavi A, et al. Assessment of age-related morpho-logical and functional changes of selected structures of the head and neck by computed tomography, magnetic resonance imaging, and positron emission tomography. Semin Nucl Med. 2007;37(2):88–102.

Medbery R, Yousem DM, Needham MF, Kligerman MM. Variation in parotid gland size, configuration, and anatomic relations. Radiother Oncol. 2000;54(1):87–9.

Prince JS, Stark P. Normal cross-sectional dimensions of the thyroid gland on routine chest CT scans. J Comput Assist Tomogr. 2002;26(3):346–8.

Raz E, Saba L, Hagiwara M, Hygino de Cruz LC Jr, Som PM, Fatterpekar GM. Parotid gland atrophy in patients with chronic trigeminal nerve denervation. AJNR Am J Neuroradiol. 2013;34(4):860–3.

Vogler RC, Ii FJ, Pilgram TK. Age-specific size of the normal adenoid pad on magnetic resonance imaging. Clin Otolaryngol Allied Sci. 2000;25(5): 392–5.

Printed in the United States
By Bookmasters